Roberto Patarca-Montero, MD, Phd, HCLD

# The Concise Encyclopedia of Fibromyalgia and Myofascial Pain

*Pre-publication*
*REVIEWS,*
*COMMENTARIES,*
*EVALUATIONS . . .*

"This encyclopedia provides the reader with a relevant and up-to-date bibliography related to fibromyalgia and myofascial pain. This is an admirable source for reference material for individuals who desire increased knowledge of either of these syndromes."

**Kimberly Groner, MSN, RN, CANP**
*Adult Nurse Practitioner,*
*Georgetown University*

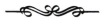

"Who would need a concise encyclopedia of fibromyalgia and myofascial pain? I would. And so would physicians, psychologists, social workers, physiotherapists, occupational therapists, and others who in their work meet people with fibromyalgia. Those engaged in patient support groups could be interested in having this encyclopedia at hand, as it is an easy way to get to the answers to the many questions that patients with fibromyalgia have. Between 'Abuse' and 'Zolpidem,' there are more than 100 entries. The selection of references, almost 800 in all, is appropriate. The relevant literature is well covered. Research on fibromyalgia is rapidly expanding, and I hope that the encyclopedia will be updated as necessary."

**Karl G. Henriksson, MD, PhD**
*Associate Professor*
*and Former Head of Neuromuscular*
*Unit and Pain Clinic,*
*University Hospital,*
*Linköping, Sweden*

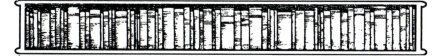

*More pre-publication*
*REVIEWS, COMMENTARIES, EVALUATIONS . . .*

"This book enables you to find specific information about fibromyalgia and myofascial pain quickly and effectively. As pathogenesis and etiology of these diseases are still poorly understood and as there is no highly effective fibromyalgia therapy, this book summarizes and presents the available knowledge.

The extensive bibliography facilitates finding the relevant original work. I recommend this book to the reader who is interested in a wide variety of topics and who seeks a better understanding of the presented disorders."

**Dieter E. Pongratz, MD**
*Professor of Internal Medicine
and Neurology,
Friedrich-Baur Institute,
University of Munich, Germany*

The Haworth Medical Press®
An Imprint of The Haworth Press, Inc.
New York • London • Oxford

# The Concise Encyclopedia
# of Fibromyalgia
# and Myofascial Pain

THE HAWORTH MEDICAL PRESS®
Chronic Fatigue Syndrome, Fibromyalgia Syndrome,
and Myalgic Encephalomyelitis

Roberto Patarca-Montero, MD, PhD
Senior Editor

*Concise Encyclopedia of Chronic Fatigue Syndrome* by Roberto Patarca-Montero

*CFIDS, Fibromyalgia, and the Virus-Allergy Link: Hidden Viruses, Allergies, and Uncommon Fatigue/Pain Disorders* by R. Bruce Duncan

*Adolescence and Myalgic Encephalomyelitis/Chronic Fatigue Syndrome: Journeys with the Dragon* by Naida Edgar Brotherston

*Phytotherapy of Chronic Fatigue Syndrome: Evidence-Based and Potentially Useful Botanicals in the Treatment of CFS* by Roberto Patarca-Montero

*Autogenic Training: A Mind-Body Approach to the Treatment of Fibromyalgia and Chronic Pain Syndrome* by Micah R. Sadigh

*Enteroviral and Toxin Mediated Myalgic Encephalomyelitis/ Chronic Fatigue Syndrome and Other Organ Pathologies* by John Richardson

*Treatment of Chronic Fatigue Syndrome in the Antiviral Revolution Era* by Roberto Patarca-Montero

*Chronic Fatigue Syndrome, Christianity, and Culture: Between God and an Illness* by James M. Rotholz

*The Concise Encyclopedia of Fibromyalgia and Myofascial Pain* by Roberto Patarca-Montero

*Chronic Fatigue Syndrome and the Body's Immune Defense System* by Roberto Patarca-Montero

# The Concise Encyclopedia of Fibromyalgia and Myofascial Pain

Roberto Patarca-Montero, MD, PhD, HCLD

The Haworth Medical Press®
An Imprint of The Haworth Press, Inc.
New York • London • Oxford

Published by

The Haworth Medical Press®, an imprint of The Haworth Press, Inc., 10 Alice Street, Binghamton, NY 13904-1580.

Cover design byAnastasia Litwak.

**Library of Congress Cataloging-in-Publication Data**

Patarca-Montero, Roberto.
    The concise encyclopedia of fibromyalgia and myofascial pain / Roberto Patarca-Montero.
        p. cm.
    Includes bibliographical references and index.
    ISBN 0-7890-1527-7 (hard : alk. paper)—ISBN 0-7890-1528-5 (soft : alk. paper)
    1. Fibromyalgia—Encyclopedias. 2. Myofascial pain syndromes—Encyclopedias. I. Title.
    [DNLM: 1. Fibromyalgia—English. 2. Myfascial Pain Syndromes—Encyclopedias—English.
    WE 13 P294c 2001]
    RC927.3 .P28 2001
    616.7'4—dc21
                                                                        2001051687

# Preface

Although much has been learned over the past decade about fibromyalgia and myofascial pain syndromes, much remains to be discovered about its causes, nosology, treatment, and overlap with a variety of rheumatic and nonrheumatic conditions. Advances in rheumatology, cardiovascular medicine, endocrinology, epidemiology, immunology, infectious disease, neurology, psychiatry, and psychology have served as the basis for the formulation of new lines of research and novel therapeutic interventions.

The purpose of this concise encyclopedia is to summarize the knowledge gained and published mainly within the past decade. The text has been organized in such a way that the reader can easily access and become familiar with the highlights of the most relevant topics. Information on particular studies involving population size and methodology is summarized to provide a framework to assess the validity and generalizability of the observations presented. The reader is encouraged to use the index to search for specific subtopics or terms that are covered under more general headings.

A balanced view is presented in each category, and the lessons learned in related disorders are also highlighted. Evidence-based alternative medicine approaches for fibromyalgia are also included in this text. It is the hope of the author that this compendium will inspire more research into the field of fibromyalgia and myofascial pain syndromes and that it will serve to educate and create greater awareness among health care professionals and the general public about these widespread problems.

# ABOUT THE AUTHOR

**Roberto Patarca-Montero, MD, PhD, HCLD,** is Assistant Professor of Medicine, Microbiology, and Immunology and also serves as Research Director of the E. M. Papper Laboratory of Clinical Immunology at the University of Miami School of Medicine. Previously, he was Assistant Professor of Pathology at the Dana-Farber Cancer Institute and Harvard Medical School in Boston. Dr. Patarca serves as Editor of *Critical Reviews in Oncogenesis* and the *Journal of Chronic Fatigue Syndrome.* He is also the author or co-author of more than 100 articles in journals or books, as well as the *Concise Encyclopedia of Chronic Fatigue Syndrome and Chronic Fatigue Syndrome: Advances in Epidemiologic, Clinical, and Basic Science Research.* He is currently conducting research on immunotherapy of AIDS and chronic fatigue syndrome. Dr. Patarca is a member of the Board of Directors of the American Association for Chronic Fatigue Syndrome and the Acquired Non-HIV Immune Diseases Foundation.

**abuse:** Anderberg et al. (2000) and Anderberg (2000) documented that stressful life events in childhood/adolescence and in adulthood seem to be very common in those who have fibromyalgia. Furthermore, these life events were experienced as more negative than the life events experienced by healthy controls. Goldberg et al. (1999) found that 64.7 percent of fibromyalgia patients studied—61.9 percent of those with myofascial pain and 50 percent of those with fascial pain—had childhood traumatic events, which are significantly related to chronic pain. Since the problem of child abuse is broad, health and rehabilitation agencies must shift from individualized treatment to interdisciplinary treatment of the family and patient.

Winfield (2000) pointed out that female gender, adverse experiences during childhood, psychological vulnerability to stress, and a stressful, often frightening environment and culture are important antecedents of fibromyalgia. Walker et al. (1997) compared thirty-six patients with fibromyalgia and thirty-three patients with rheumatoid arthritis and found that those with fibromyalgia had significantly higher lifetime prevalence rates of all forms of victimization, both adult and childhood, as well as combinations of adult and childhood trauma. Although childhood maltreatment was found to be a general risk factor for fibromyalgia, particular forms of maltreatment (e.g., sexual abuse per se) did not have specific effects. Experiences of physical assault in adulthood, however, showed a strong and specific relationship with unexplained pain. Trauma severity was correlated significantly with measures of physical disability, psychiatric distress, illness adjustment, personality, and quality of sleep in patients with fibromyalgia but not in those with rheumatoid arthritis.

In a study of seventy-five women with fibromyalgia, 57 percent of whom had a history of abuse, Alexander et al. (1998) reported an association between sexual/physical abuse and increased use of outpatient health care services and medications for pain. Abused patients also were characterized by significantly greater pain, fatigue, functional disability, and stress, as well as by a tendency to label dolorimeter stimuli as painful regardless of their intensities. Finestone et al. (2000) also found that women with a history of childhood sexual abuse reported more chronic pain symptoms and utilized more health care resources than nonabused control subjects.

*1*

**acupuncture:** There are various acupuncture techniques and methods, including dry needling, electroacupuncture, acupuncture using hypodermic needles, and injecting various solutions into the acupuncture sites (reviewed in Ridgway, 1999). Several review and meta-analysis papers on clinical trials (Berman et al., 1999, 2000; Koenig and Stevermer, 1999; Lee, 2000; Muller et al., 2000; Offenbacher and Stucki, 2000; Ridgway, 1999; White, 1995) as well as NIH Consensus Conferences (Acupuncture, 1997; NIH Consensus Conference, 1998) have found that although acupuncture as a therapeutic intervention is widely practiced in the United States and there have been numerous studies regarding its potential usefulness, many of these studies provide equivocal results because of design, sample size, and other factors. The issue is further complicated by inherent difficulties in the use of appropriate controls, such as placebos and sham acupuncture groups. However, promising results have emerged, for example, showing efficacy of acupuncture as treatment for adult postoperative and chemotherapy nausea and vomiting and for postoperative dental pain. There are other situations, such as addiction, stroke rehabilitation, headache, menstrual cramps, tennis elbow, fibromyalgia, myofascial pain, osteoarthritis, lower back pain, carpal tunnel syndrome, and asthma, in which acupuncture may be useful as an adjunct treatment or as an acceptable alternative; or it may be included in a comprehensive management program.

Basic science research has demonstrated convincingly that, at least in the context of acute pain, acupuncture's effects are related to the release of a variety of natural opioids. For instance, in a study of twenty-nine fibromyalgia patients, Sprott et al. (1998) reported that acupuncture treatment was associated with decreased pain levels, fewer positive tender points, decreased serotonin concentration in platelets, an increase of the serum levels of the pain-modulating substances serotonin and substance P, and improved microcirculation in tender points. Ridgway (1999) also reported that acupuncture is effective for the treatment of a type of chronic back pain that is possibly associated with a radiculopathically induced, hypersensitivity myofascial syndrome that presents as a fibromyalgia-like syndrome. A high-quality study found that real acupuncture is more effective than sham acupuncture for relieving pain, increasing pain thresholds, improving global ratings, and reducing morning stiffness of fibromyalgia (reviewed in Berman et al., 1999). Electroacupuncture may also be useful in the treatment of fibromyalgia (White, 1995). However, it should be noted that for some fibromyalgia patients, acupuncture can exacerbate symptoms, further complicating its application for this condition (Berman and Swyers, 1999).

**affective distress and anxiety:** A study in Germany by Walter et al. (1998) comparing low back pain patients with and without fibromyalgia syndrome (15 and 120 patients, respectively) found that although fibromyalgia patients showed remarkably higher levels of pain severity and affective distress, these pronounced differences disappeared after controlling for different levels of pain severity. The authors concluded that affective distress is not a unique feature of fibromyalgia but seems to be caused entirely by higher levels of pain severity.

Wolfe and Skevington (2000) reported that fibromyalgia patients suffered more distress in association with increased functional impairment as compared to rheumatoid arthritis or osteoarthritis patients. Hallberg and Carlsson (1998) also found that fibromyalgia patients scored significantly higher on trait anxiety and seemed to interpret stressful situations as more threatening than did patients with work-related muscular pain. Anxiety seems to be of central importance for coping with chronic pain, and anxiety-prone patients with fibromyalgia might benefit from psychological support in the process of coping with pain (Hallberg and Carlsson, 1998).

Celiker et al. (1997) suggest that current anxiety is not secondary to pain but trait anxiety is possibly causally related to pain in fibromyalgia. Studies by Kurtze et al. (1998, 1999) of 322 fibromyalgia patients found independent, additive effects of anxiety and depression upon levels of pain and fatigue. Whereas interaction between anxiety and depression failed to significantly explain pain and fatigue symptom differences among the participants, it significantly affected quality of life, functional disability, and lifestyle and was associated with high consumption of coffee and cigarettes. The finding that anxiety and depression are independently associated with severity of pain symptoms in fibromyalgia is underscored by the study by Fischler et al. (1997) which failed to find marked differences in illness-related features or in psychiatric morbidity between CFS patients with and without fibromyalgia.

**aging and geriatrics:** The prevalence of fibromyalgia increases with age (Buckwalter and Lappin, 2000; Goldenberg, 1996). Neck pain, joint pain, and fibromyalgia all appear to increase with age in both genders, whereas abdominal pain and tension-type headaches decrease with age, and migraine headache and temporomandibular disorder appear to peak in the reproductive years (Meisler, 1999).

Fibromyalgia and polymyalgia rheumatica are the most common diffuse pain syndromes in the elderly (Belilos and Carsons, 1998; Gowin, 2000). Fibromyalgia may be a primary or a secondary phenomenon of other diffuse pain syndromes associated with inflammatory, endocrine, or neoplastic diseases (Gowin, 2000). The initial manifestations of fibromyalgia and other rheumatologic disorders in elderly patients may differ from the typical findings in younger patients. Geriatric patients may have nonspecific complaints, a decline in physical function, or even confusion. Common soft tissue problems encountered in older adults, including fibromyalgia, selected bursitis/tendinitis syndromes, nerve entrapment syndromes, and miscellaneous manifestations such as Dupuytren's contractures, trigger fingers, palmar fasciitis, and reflex-sympathetic dystrophy are generally diagnosed as arthritis or normal age-related problems but need to be distinguished clinically (Holland and Gonzalez, 1998). In the selection of optimal pharmacologic and nonpharmacologic therapeutic modalities in the geriatric population, clinicians should focus on maintaining or improving the patient's quality of life and level of independent function (Michet et al., 1995).

**alcohol:** Alcohol consumption may exacerbate symptomatology in fibromyalgia (Eisinger, 1998).

**allergy:** Tuncer et al. (1997) reported a high frequency of allergy background among thirty-two primary fibromyalgia patients when compared with an age- and sex-matched control group. Allergic skin tests, which could not be performed in the control group, were positive in ten of fifteen primary fibromyalgia patients. Although serum IgE levels were found elevated in the primary fibromyalgia group, the elevation was not statistically significant (Tuncer et al., 1997).

**aloe:** One study showed that freeze-dried *Aloe vera* gel extract or a combination of freeze-dried *Aloe vera* gel extract and additional plant-derived saccharides resulted in a remarkable reduction in initial symptom severity among fifty patients with chronic fatigue syndrome and fibromyalgia, with continued improvement in the nine-month period between initial assessment and follow-up (Dykman et al., 1998). Aloe plants are native to eastern and southern Africa. Gel from the inner central zone of the leaves and latex from pericyclic cells are used for medicinal purposes. Primary active components include anthraquinones, saccharides, prostaglandins, and fatty acids (Hadley and Petry, 1999).

**alternative and complementary medicine:** Fibromyalgia is a chronic-pain–related syndrome associated with high rates (approximately two-thirds of patients in most studies) of complementary and alternative medicine use, usually concomitant with multiple interventions (Berman and Swyers, 1997, 1999; Dimmock et al., 1996; Hawkins, 1998; Nicassio et al., 1997; Pioro-Boisset et al., 1996; Rao et al., 1999). Factors associated with alternative and complementary medicine use include high socioeconomic status, duration of fibromyalgia, and dissatisfaction with current hospital treatment (Dimmock et al., 1996). The relatively high cost of and lack of information on complementary therapies appears to dissuade those patients who choose not to use it (Dimmock et al., 1996). Moreover, based on a study of eighty-two fibromyalgia patients, Fitzcharles and Esdaile (1997) found that patients who had been treated by nonphysician practitioners during the preceding six months reported similar pain and functional impairment to those not receiving treatments.

Among the many alternative and complementary medicine therapies frequently used by fibromyalgia patients, empirical research data exist to support the use of only three (in order of strength of supporting data): (1) mind-body techniques (e.g., biofeedback, hypnosis, and cognitive-behavioral therapy, particularly when utilized as part of a multidisciplinary approach to treatment), (2) acupuncture, and (3) manipulative therapies (e.g., chiropractic and massage) (Berman and Swyers, 1999). (*See* BIOFEEDBACK, HYPNOSIS, COGNITIVE-BEHAVIORAL THERAPY, ACUPUNCTURE, CHIROPRACTIC TREATMENT, and MASSAGE for details of each). However, in one study (Pioro-Boisset et al., 1996), patient satisfaction ratings were highest for spiritual interventions.

**amitriptyline:** Amitriptyline is a tricyclic antidepressant agent that also has analgesic properties (Bryson and Wilde, 1996). Whether amitriptyline's analgesic effects are linked to its mood-altering activity or attributable to a discrete pharmacological action (or a combination of both) is unknown. Clinical trials demonstrate that oral amitriptyline achieves at least a good or moderate response in up to two-thirds of patients with postherpetic neuralgia and three-quarters of patients with painful diabetic neuropathy, which are neurogenic pain syndromes that are often unresponsive to narcotic analgesics (Godfrey, 1996; Johnson, 1997).

Amitriptyline has also demonstrated efficacy in heterogeneous groups of patients with chronic nonmalignant pain, such as that encountered in fibromyalgia. In this respect, a four-center, twelve-week study of 130 female fibromyalgia patients not suffering from psychiatric disorders showed that 74 percent responded to amitriptyline (25-37.5 mg/day) and managed best in general health, pain, sleep quality and quantity, and fatigue (Hannonen et al., 1998). In terms of nonresponders to amitriptyline, a study of twenty-two fibromyalgia patients in a two-month, double-blind, crossover trial of amitriptyline (25 mg/day) versus placebo found that an anomaly consisting of electroencephalographic waves within the alpha frequency band during non–rapid-eye movement sleep, which is present in only a small proportion of patients with fibromyalgia and does not correlate with disease severity, is not affected by treatment with amitriptyline (Carette et al., 1995). A larger sample size will be needed to adequately assess the value of this sleep anomaly in predicting the response to amitriptyline.

Adverse events resulting from the antimuscarinic activity of amitriptyline (primarily dry mouth and sedation) are commonly reported, even at the low dosages used for the control of pain (Lautenschlager, 2000). Low starting doses and careful dosage titration may help to minimize these effects. Orthostatic hypotension and tachycardia, sometimes associated with tricyclic antidepressant agents, may also pose a problem in the elderly.

**anticardiolipin antibody:** Anticardiolipin antibodies occur in a wide variety of autoimmune and nonautoimmune disorders in adults. A study of 106 pediatric patients (36 systemic lupus erythematosus, 28 juvenile rheumatoid arthritis, 11 fibromyalgia, 7 sarcoidosis, 5 dermatomyositis, 3 rheumatic fever, 3 vasculitis, 2 scleroderma, and 11 miscellaneous) failed to find anticardiolipin antibodies or features of antiphospholipid syndrome among pediatric fibromyalgia patients (Gedalia et al., 1998).

**antidepressants:** O'Malley et al. (2000) performed a meta-analysis of published English-language, randomized, placebo-controlled trials (sixteen identified, thirteen of which were deemed appropriate for data extraction) and concluded that antidepressants, regardless of class (three assessed: tricyclics, selective serotonin reuptake inhibitors, and S-adenosylmethionine), are efficacious in treating many symptoms of fibromyalgia (sleep, fatigue, pain, and well-being, but not trigger points). Patients were more than four times as likely to report overall improvement, and reported moderate reductions in individual symptoms, particularly pain. In the five studies where there was adequate assessment for an effect independent of depression, only one study found a correlation between symptom improvement and depression scores. Whether this effect is independent of depression needs further study. A previous meta-analysis by O'Malley et al. (1999) had arrived at similar conclusions. Arnold et al. (2000) also reviewed twenty-one randomized, controlled clinical trials, identified sixteen involving tricyclic agents, and performed meta-analysis with the nine of the sixteen studies that were considered suitable. Compared with placebo, tricyclic agents were associated with effect sizes that were substantially larger than zero for all measurements of physician and patient overall assessment, pain, stiffness, tenderness, fatigue, and sleep quality. The largest improvement was associated with measures of sleep quality; the most modest improvement was found in measures of stiffness and tenderness. Other review articles suggest that antidepressants play an important role in the drug treatment of chronic pain and fibromyalgia (Baraczka et al., 1997; Fishbain, 2000; Godfrey, 1996; Johnson, 1997; Lautenschlager, 2000; Maes et al., 1999; Touchon, 1995). However, moclobemide, a reversible inhibitor of monoamine oxidase, seems to be ineffective and inferior to amitriptyline for pain (Hannonen et al., 1998).

**antiganglioside antibodies:** Klein and Berg (1995) reported a defined autoantibody pattern consisting of antibodies directed against serotonin, gangliosides, and phospholipids in about 70 percent of fibromyalgia patients and in about 55 percent of chronic fatigue syndrome patients. Although 71 percent of 100 fibromyalgia patients and 43 percent of forty-two chronic fatigue syndrome patients studied had antiganglioside antibodies, antibodies directed against gangliosides and phospholipids could also be detected in other disorders, while the presence of antiserotonin antibodies seemed more closely related to fibromyalgia and chronic fatigue syndrome. The observation that family members of fibromyalgia and chronic fatigue syndrome patients also had these antibodies represents an argument in favor of a genetic predisposition (*see* GENETICS).

**antinuclear antibodies:** A study by Suarez-Almazor et al. (1998) of 711 patients showed that primary care physicians frequently requested antinuclear antibodies (ANA), rheumatoid factor, and erythrocyte sedimentation rate in patients referred to rheumatologists. Most tests were negative and were often requested in patients without connective tissue diseases, resulting in low positive predictive values and questionable clinical utility. Suarez-Almazor et al. (1998) suggest that a decrease in inappropriate use could be achieved by emphasizing that fatigue and diffuse musculoskeletal pain are not indicative of connective tissue disease in the absence of other features such as joint swelling, typical rash, or organ involvement. In fact, most patients with diffuse musculoskeletal pain and fatigue in their study had fibromyalgia or localized soft tissue rheumatism. Based on a study performed by fifteen international laboratories, Tan et al. (1997) recommend that laboratories performing immunofluorescent ANA tests should report results at both the 1:40 and 1:160 dilutions and should supply information on the percentage of normal individuals who are positive at these dilutions, because a low-titer ANA is not necessarily insignificant. ANA assays can be a useful discriminant in recognizing certain disease conditions, but can create misunderstanding when the limitations are not fully appreciated (Illei and Klippel, 1999).

**antiphospholipid antibodies:** Berg et al. (1999) found low level coagulation activation from immunoglobulins, as demonstrated by anti-B2GPI antibodies, in patients with fibromyalgia or chronic fatigue syndrome, a finding that, according to Berg et al., would allow classification of these diseases as a type of antiphospholipid antibody syndrome. However, Gedalia et al. (1998) found no evidence of antiphospholipid antibody syndrome among pediatric fibromyalgia patients. Although antiphospholipid antibodies can be found in disorders other than fibromyalgia, Klein and Berg (1995) reported an increased frequency of antiphospholipid antibodies in conjunction with antigangliosides or antiserotonin antibodies among fibromyalgia or chronic fatigue syndrome patients. Heller et al. (1998) also found the latter autoantibody pattern among patients with sudden deafness and progressive hearing loss, a significant proportion of whom also complained of fatigue, myalgia, arthralgia, depression, diarrhea, and sicca symptoms.

**antipolymer antibodies:** Wilson et al. (1999) found a higher seroprevalence of antipolymer antibodies in patients with fibromyalgia (22/47, 47 percent) compared to patients with osteoarthritis (3/16, 19 percent) or rheumatoid arthritis (1/13, 8 percent), as well as compared to banked autoimmune disease control sera from patients with poly/dermatomyosis (2/15, 13 percent), rheumatoid arthritis (3/30, 10 percent), systemic lupus erythematosus (1/30, 3 percent), and systemic sclerosis (1/30, 3 percent). The prevalence of antipolymer antibody seroreactivity was also significantly higher in patients with severe fibromyalgia (17/28, 61 percent) compared to patients with mild fibromyalgia (11/37, 30 percent) and controls (4/21, 19 percent). In addition, both mean threshold and mean tolerance dolorimetry scores were significantly lower in the antipolymer antibody seropositive patients with mild fibromyalgia compared to the seronegative patients. Wilson et al. (1999) suggest that the antipolymer antibody assay may be an objective marker in the diagnosis and assessment of fibromyalgia and may provide additional avenues of investigation into the pathophysiological processes involved in fibromyalgia, whether primary or secondary to other disease processes, such as that associated with silicone breast implantation (Angell, 1997; Edlavitch, 1997; Ellis et al., 1997; Everson and Blackburn, 1997; Korn, 1997; Lamm, 1997).

**antiserotonin antibodies:** Klein and Berg (1995) showed the presence of a defined autoantibody pattern consisting of antiserotonin, antiphospholipid, and antigangliosides antibodies in approximately 70 percent of fibromyalgia patients and 50 percent of chronic fatigue syndrome patients. Antiserotonin antibodies were closely related with fibromyalgia/chronic fatigue syndrome, while antiganglioside and antiphospholipid antibodies could also be detected in other disorders. Olin et al. (1998) confirmed the latter findings. Heller et al. (1998) found a similar pattern of autoantibody reactivity in patients with sudden deafness or progressive hearing loss who complained of symptoms typical for fibromyalgia/chronic fatigue syndrome, while Coplan et al. (1999) also found a significant prevalence of anti-serotonin antibodies among patients with panic disorder. It remains to be demonstrated if the peripheral autoimmunity is representative of central nervous system serotonin neuronal alterations (Neeck et al., 1996).

**artists and musicians:** Martinez-Lavin et al. (2000) reported on the influence of fibromyalgia in Frida Kahlo's life and art. The two great pianists Clara Wieck Schumann (1819-1896) and Sergei Vassilievich Rachmaninov (1873-1943) suffered from chronic pain, and a report by Hingtgen (1999) discusses the pain syndromes that plagued these great musicians and the effect of chronic illness on their music. It is important for the physician to differentiate fibromyalgia from the pain, sensory loss, and lack of coordination that may result from the physical demands of performing on musical instruments (Potter and Jones, 1995).

**ascorbigen:** In a one-month open-label trial, Bramwell et al. (2000) gave 500 mg per day of a blend containing 100 mg ascorbigen and 400 mg broccoli powder to twelve female fibromyalgia patients. Patients showed a mean decrease in their physical impairment score and total fibromyalgia impact scores and an increase in the mean threshold pain level. However, the mean physical impairment score two weeks posttreatment showed a significant return to near pretreatment level, and a larger, double-blind study is needed.

**attributions:** Neerinckx et al. (2000) found that the majority of patients with chronic fatigue syndrome and fibromyalgia reported a great diversity of attributions ("a chemical imbalance in my body," "a virus," "stress," and "emotional confusion") open to a preferably personalized cognitive-behavioral approach. Neerinckx et al. (2000) recommend paying special attention to patients with symptoms existing for more than one year and to those who had previous contact

with a self-help group because they particularly show external, sta-
ble, and global attributions that may compromise feelings of self-efficacy in dealing with the illness.

**autoimmune fatigue syndrome:** Itoh et al. (1997) found that among
children who chronically complain of nonspecific symptoms such as
headache, fatigue, abdominal pain, and low-grade fever, those who
were antinuclear antibody (ANA) positive (approximately 50 percent
of cases) tended to have general fatigue and low-grade fever, while
gastrointestinal problems, such as abdominal pain, diarrhea, and
orthostatic dysregulation symptoms, were commonly seen in ANA-
negative patients. Children who were unable to go to school more
than one day a week were seen significantly more among ANA-positive patients than among negative patients. Based on these observations, the authors concluded that autoimmunity may play a role in
childhood chronic nonspecific symptoms and proposed a new disease
entity: the autoimmune fatigue syndrome in children.

Itoh et al. (1999) described two patients with fibromyalgia who
had been diagnosed initially as having autoimmune fatigue syndrome
(AIFS) and proposed that ANA-positive fibromyalgia or ANA-positive chronic fatigue syndrome could be forms of AIFS. Itoh et al.
(1998) also reported that a novel autoantibody to a 62 kD protein
(anti-Sa) was found in 40 percent of ANA-positive children with
autoimmune fatigue syndrome. Similar to studies of autoimmune
diseases, Itoh et al. (2000) found that autoimmune fatigue syndrome
has an immunogenetic background: it is positively associated with
the class I antigen HLA-B61 and with the class II antigen HLA-DR9,
and negatively associated with HLA-DR2.

**autonomic dysfunction:** Power spectrum analyses of heart rate variability have revealed that the basal autonomic state of fibromyalgia
patients is characterized by increased sympathetic and decreased
parasympathetic tones (Cohen et al., 2000) and a deranged sympathetic response to orthostatic stress (Kelemen et al., 1998; Martinez-
Lavin, 1997; Martinez-Lavin and Hermosillo, 2000). As is the case
with chronic fatigue syndrome (Wilke et al., 1998), Bou-Holaigah
et al. (1997) identified a strong association between fibromyalgia and
neurally mediated hypotension: During stage one of upright tilt,
twelve of twenty fibromyalgia patients (60 percent), but no controls,

had an abnormal drop in blood pressure; and among those with fibromyalgia, all eighteen who tolerated upright tilt for more than ten minutes reported worsening or provocation of their typical widespread fibromyalgia pain during stage one, while controls were asymptomatic (Bou-Holaigah et al., 1997). Individuals with fibromyalgia also have diminished twenty-four-hour heart rate variability due to an increased nocturnal predominance of the low-frequency band oscillations consistent with an exaggerated sympathetic modulation of the sinus node (Martinez-Lavin et al., 1998). This abnormal chronobiology could explain the sleep disturbances and fatigue that occur in this syndrome. Spectral analysis of heart rate variability may therefore be a useful test to identify fibromyalgia patients who have dysautonomia.

The autonomic nervous system is a major mediator of the visceral response to central influences such as psychological stress, and autonomic dysfunction may also represent the physiological pathway accounting for many of the extraintestinal symptoms seen in irritable bowel syndrome patients and some of the frequent gastrointestinal complaints reported by patients with disorders, such as chronic fatigue and fibromyalgia (Tougas, 1999). However, sympathetic dysautonomia may present differentially among the latter syndromes since denervation hypersensitivity of the pupil is not apparent in chronic fatigue syndrome patients (Sendrowski et al., 1997).

**B**

**Behcet's syndrome:** Yavuz et al. (1998) found a trend for an increased frequency of fibromyalgia in female Behcet's syndrome patients. In their study, ten (nine of whom were women) of 108 Behcet's syndrome patients (9.2 percent) met the American College of Rheumatology criteria for fibromyalgia, and, in contrast to those without fibromyalgia, they had mild to moderate disease activity in which musculoskeletal complaints were common.

**benzodiazepine-induced hip fracture:** Fibromyalgia patients on long-acting benzodiazepines may be at increased risk for osteoporosis and hip fracture (Robb-Nicholson, 1998).

**biofeedback:** Based on a study of nineteen fibromyalgia patients, Mur et al. (1999) concluded that electromyography-based (EMG) biofeedback training may contribute not only to a reduction of pain and muscle tension but also to improvement of quality of life. The latter results are consistent with a previous study of eighteen patients by Sarnoch et al. (1997), and Mur et al. recommend EMG biofeedback as part of a multimodal pain therapy in fibromyalgia patients. In this respect, Buckelew et al. (1998) randomized 199 fibromyalgia patients to four groups: biofeedback/relaxation, exercise, a combined program of the latter two, and an educational/attention control program. All three treatment interventions resulted in improved self-efficacy for physical function which was best maintained by the combination group after a two-year follow-up period.

**Borna disease virus:** Borna disease virus is a neurotropic RNA virus that gives rise to a characteristic pathological picture described as meningoencephalomyelitis in horses and sheep. Epidemiological data suggest that Borna disease virus may be closely associated with neuropsychiatric disease (depression and schizophrenia) in humans. Furthermore, anti-Borna disease virus antibodies and Borna disease virus RNA was detected in a family cluster with chronic fatigue syndrome (Kitani et al., 1996; Nakaya et al., 1996, 1997). However, a study of eighteen Danish patients with fibromyalgia failed to reveal Borna disease virus in cerebrospinal fluid or serum (Wittrup et al., 2000).

**botulinum toxin:** Paulson and Gill (1996) reported that, unlike the case for migraine headaches, botulinum toxin is unsatisfactory therapy for fibromyalgia.

**breast implants:** Although some authors in older studies have suggested a link with fibromyalgia or soft tissue rheumatism (Bridges et al., 1996; Cuellar et al., 1995; Fuchs et al., 1995; Levenson et al., 1996; Vasey, 1997; Vasey and Aziz, 1995; Young et al., 1995), immunologic and other sequelae of silicone breast implantation such as collagen vascular diseases or fibromyalgia have not been confirmed in large studies and reviews (Blackburn et al., 1997; Brown et al., 1998; Friis et al., 1997; Lai et al., 2000; Levine et al., 2000; Martin,

1999; Nyren et al., 1998; Peters et al., 1997; Thomas et al., 1997; Wolfe, 1999; Wolfe and Anderson, 1999). Several reports have discussed the possible silicone breast implant-associated induction of autoimmunity, in particular antipolymer antibodies whose presence has also been reported in fibromyalgia (Angell, 1997; Edlavitch, 1997; Ellis et al., 1997; Everson and Blackburn, 1997; Korn, 1997; Lamm, 1997; Romano, 1996; Silverman et al., 1996). However, many studies have failed to find evidence for autoimmunity or other immunological abnormalities. For instance, Blackburn et al. (1997) found that the levels of interleukin-6, interleukin-8, tumor necrosis factor-alpha, soluble intercellular adhesion molecule-1, and soluble interleukin-2 receptor were not different in silicone breast implant disease patients from those seen in normal subjects and were significantly less than those seen when examining chronic inflammatory disorders such as rheumatoid arthritis or systemic lupus erythematosus. Although Young et al. (1995) found a higher frequency of HLA-DR53 among symptomatic breast implant patients and Bridges et al. (1996) reported 5 percent positivity for antinuclear antibodies among silicone breast implant patients, these findings have not panned out in larger analyses. Nonetheless, some studies have found that breast implants appear to be more common in patients with fibromyalgia than in those without it, an observation that has led some authors to postulate that there may be a common, predisposing set of psychosocial characteristics that are shared between those who have fibromyalgia and those who undergo silicone breast implantation (Wolfe and Anderson, 1999).

Although uncontrolled case series have reported neurologic problems believed to be associated with silicone breast implants, one review report (Rosenberg, 1996) failed to find any evidence that silicone breast implants are causally related to the development of any neurologic diseases. The latter study found that although neurologic symptoms were frequently endorsed, including fatigue (82 percent), memory loss and other cognitive impairment (76 percent), and generalized myalgias (66 percent), most patients (66 percent) had normal neurological examinations. Findings reported as abnormal were mild and usually subjective, including sensory abnormalities in 23 percent, mental status abnormalities in 13 percent, and reflex changes in 8 percent. No pattern of laboratory abnormalities was seen, either in combination or in attempts to correlate them with the clinical situation. Laboratory studies appeared to be random without an attempt to confirm or correlate with a particular diagnosis. Diagnoses by physicians endorsing the concept that silicone breast implants (SBIs) cause illness included "human adjuvant disease" in all cases, memory loss and other cognitive impairment ("silicone encephalopathy") and/or "atypical neurologic disease syndrome" in 73 percent, "atypical neurologic multiple sclerosis-like syndrome" in 8 percent, chronic inflammatory demyelinating polyneuropathy in 23 percent, and some other type of peripheral neuropathy in 18 percent. There was no coherence in making these diagnoses; the presence of any symptoms in these women was sufficient to make these diagnoses. Alternatively, after review of the data, no neurologic diagnosis could be made in 82 percent. Neurologic symptoms could be explained in some cases by depression ($n = 16$), fibromyalgia ($n = 9$), radiculopathy ($n = 7$), anxiety disorders ($n = 4$), multiple sclerosis ($n = 4$), multifocal motor neuropathy ($n = 1$), carpal tunnel syndrome ($n = 1$), dermatomyositis ($n = 1$), and other psychiatric disorders ($n = 3$).

**breathing:** In a study of seventeen fibromyalgia patients, Sergi et al. (1999) found that the respiratory pattern of fibromyalgia patients showed a high occurrence of periodic breathing, a greater number of desaturations per hour of sleep, and a lower transfer factor of the lung for carbon monoxide despite no changes in pulmonary volumes. The transfer factor for carbon monoxide was more impaired and the occurrence of periodic breathing was higher among patients complaining of daytime hypersomnolence who had a higher number of tender points, about twice as many arousals per hour and a lower sleep efficiency than patients who did not report this symptom. Other studies have shown changes in sleep respiratory patterns of fibromyalgia patients (Alvarez-Lario and Viejo Banuelos, 1997), and Ozgocmen and Ardicoglu (1999) reported reduced chest expansion in primary fibromyalgia syndrome. Weiss et al. (1998) described two patients with chronic, severe, episodic dyspnea who underwent prolonged, extensive, and invasive evaluations without a diagnosis being made and were both subsequently diagnosed with fibromyalgia. The latter authors point out that fibromyalgia is rarely included in the differential diagnosis of dyspnea, and timely diagnosis and treatment may be delayed.

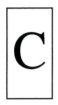 **calcitonin:** In a double-blind crossover trial in which eleven fibromyalgia patients alternatively received salmon calcitonin (100 IU s.c.) and isotonic saline (1 cc s.c.) for four weeks, with a four-week washout period between treatments, none of the eleven outcomes measures showed a significant improvement, an observation that suggests that subcutaneous calcitonin injection is not effective in the treatment of fibromyalgia (Bessette et al. 1998.).

**cancer chemotherapy:** In a study by Warner et al. (1997), of eight women with no previous rheumatic history, four developed polyarthritis (one seropositive), three fibromyalgia, and one spondylosis after the diagnosis and during or after treatment of breast cancer. Of fifteen women with breast cancer who had previous rheumatic symptoms, twelve developed worse and/or new symptoms after chemotherapy. In both groups, the symptoms had a significant negative impact on functional status, and in some cases resolution was only partial even after many years of follow-up. Warner et al. (1997) suggest that prospective studies are needed to determine the incidence, risk factors, and optimal management of fibromyalgia or nondestructive polyarthropathy in women who receive systemic adjuvant therapy for breast cancer. Some chemotherapeutic agents, such as tamoxifen, may help relieve fibromyalgia symptoms (Simonson, 1996).

**carpal tunnel syndrome:** An association between fibromyalgia and carpal tunnel syndrome has been reported (Cimmino et al., 1996; Perez-Ruiz et al., 1997) and, in a study of 100 cases, Straub (1999) identified fibromyalgia and myofascial pain syndrome as preoperative factors associated with an increased likelihood of unsatisfactory results from endoscopic carpal tunnel release.

**chemical intolerance:** Several studies indicate that low level chemical intolerance (CI) is a symptom of several different chronic and sometimes overlapping conditions in which women are over-represented, such as fibromyalgia, chronic fatigue syndrome, multiple chemical sensitivity, sick building syndrome, and Persian Gulf War syndrome (Bell, Baldwin, Russek, et al., 1998; Bell, Baldwin, and Schwartz, 1998; Bell et al., 1999; Csef, 1998; Fiedler et al., 1996; Gibson et al., 1998; Lohmann et al., 1996; "Multiple Chemical Sensitivity: A 1999 Consensus," 1999; Slotkoff et al., 1997; Weiss, 1998). Severe CI is a characteristic of 20 to 47 percent of individuals with apparent fibromyalgia and/or chronic fatigue syndrome, all patients with multiple chemical sensitivity syndrome, and approximately 4 to 6 percent of the general population (Bell, Baldwin, Russek, et al., 1998; Bell, Baldwin, and Schwartz, 1998; Bell et al., 1999; Slotkoff et al., 1997). In the general population, 15 to 30 percent report at least minor problems with CI.

Agents whose exposures are associated with symptoms and suspected of causing onset of chemical intolerance with chronic illness include gasoline, kerosene, natural gas, pesticides (especially chlordane and chlorpyrifos), solvents, new carpet and other renovation materials, adhesives/glues, fiberglass, carbonless copy paper, fabric softener, formaldehyde and glutaraldehyde, carpet shampoos (lauryl sulfate) and other cleaning agents, isocyanates, combustion products (poorly vented gas heaters, overheated batteries), and medications (dinitrochlorobenzene for warts, intranasally packed neosynephrine, prolonged antibiotics, and general anesthesia with petrochemicals). Disorders commonly seen in chemical intolerance patients are mainly nonspecific and include headache (often migraine), chronic fatigue, musculoskeletal aching, chronic respiratory inflammation (rhinitis, sinusitis, laryngitis, asthma), attention deficit, and hyperactivity (in affected younger children). Less common disorders include tremor, seizures, and mitral valve prolapse (Ziem and McTamney, 1997).

Although the levels of chemicals reported to trigger CI would normally be considered nontoxic or subtoxic, host factors may contribute to generating a disabling intensity to the resultant multisystem dysfunctions in CI (Bell, Baldwin, Russek, et al., 1998; Bell, Baldwin, and Schwartz, 1998; Bell et al., 1999; Rowat, 1999). Explanatory mechanisms of chemical intolerance include psychiatric diagnoses such as somatization (CI had strong positive correlations between serum neopterin levels and all of the scales measuring somatization) (Bell, Patarca, et al., 1998), behavioral mechanisms, such as conditioning and generalization, neuropharmacological mechanisms, such as kindling and time-dependent sensitization (including an olfactory-limbic and/or mesolimbic neural sensitization model for intolerance to low-level chemicals in the environment) (Bell, Baldwin, Russek, et al., 1998; Bell, Baldwin, and Schwartz, 1998; Bell et al., 1999), impaired porphyrin metabolism (multiple organs), and psychoneuroimmunological mechanisms, such as neurogenic inflammation (respiratory, gastrointestinal, genitourinary) and those involving the hypothalamic-pituitary-adrenal axis (Ziem and McTamney, 1997). Laboratory animal experimentation and controlled clinical trials, especially with inhaled material, provide the means for exploring the proffered explanations. In a study of cell-mediated sensitivity to environmental chemicals in thirty-nine fibromyalgia patients, Shanklin et al. (2000) found significantly higher lymphocyte proliferation indexes in response to aluminum, lead, and platinum and borderline higher to cadmium and silicon. However, fibromyalgia patients showed sporadic responses to the specific substances tested, with no high-frequency result. Miller (1999) proposed that fibromyalgia and other related conditions may be secondary to "toxicant-induced loss of tolerance," a two-step disease process in which (1) certain chemical exposures, e.g., indoor air contaminants, chemical spills, or pesticide applications, cause certain susceptible persons to lose their prior natural tolerance for common chemicals, foods, and drugs (initiation); (2) subsequently, previously tolerated exposures trigger symptoms.

**Chiari malformation:** Muller et al. (1998) point out that disturbances of posture of the vertebral column are frequently found in fibromyalgia as well as in low back pain patients. Also, reduction in the mobility of the whole spine and localized movement impairments are present in both conditions. It is likely that the disturbances are responsible for the first manifestations of fibromyalgia in a single localization, especially in lumbar and cervical regions. A particular defect in the vertebral column at the cervical level which causes partial compression of the spinal cord, the Chiari malformation, has been proposed to play an etiologic role in fibromyalgia, but compelling evidence remains elusive (Bradley and Alarcon, 1999). The latter condition is diagnosed radiologically and treated surgically.

**chiropractic treatment:** In a preliminary study, Hains and Hains (2000) found that nine of fifteen female fibromyalgia patients responded to a regimen of thirty chiropractic treatments that effectively combine ischemic compression and spinal manipulation. Reductions in pain intensity, sleep disturbance, and fatigue associated with fibro-myalgia were apparent. A trend, determined as statistically insignificant, suggests that older subjects with severe and more chronic pain and a greater number of tender points responded more poorly to treatment. Other preliminary studies have suggested efficacy of chiropratic management in the treatment of fibromyalgia (Blunt et al., 1997; Harper and Liu, 1998; Schneider, 1998).

**chlamydia:** Although it has been proposed that infection with chlamydia may be an etiologic factor for chronic fatigue syndrome and fibromyalgia, this contention needs epidemiogical and serologic substantiation because evidence of infection appears to be nonspecific (Machtey, 1997).

*Chlorella pyrenoidosa:* The results of a pilot study of eighteen fibro-myalgia patients suggest that adding daily for two months nutritional supplements derived from the unicellular green alga, *Chlorella pyrenoidosa* (10 g of "Sun Chlorella" tablets and 100 mL of liquid "Wakasa Gold"), results in a statistically significant improvement in average tender point index (Merchant et al., 2000). Seven patients felt that the dietary supplement had improved their fibromyalgia symptoms, while six thought they had experienced no change, and five believed the symptoms had worsened over the time of the trial. A larger, more comprehensive, double-blind, placebo-controlled clinical trial is needed.

**chronic fatigue syndrome:** Despite remarkably different diagnostic criteria, fibromyalgia and chronic fatigue syndrome have many demographic and clinical similarities (Bazelmans et al., 1999; Buchwald, 1996; Buchwald, Umali, et al., 1996; Clauw and Chrousos, 1997; Demitrack, 1998; Hoffmann et al., 1996; Kenner, 1998; Lloyd, 1998; White et al., 2000; Ziem and Donnay, 1995). More specifically, few differences exist in the domains of symptoms, examination findings, laboratory tests, functional status, psychosocial features, and psychiatric disorders. Among the differences between the two syndromes, Evengard et al. (1998) found that although substance P levels were normal in the cerebrospinal fluid of fifteen patients with chronic fatigue syndrome, the majority of fibromyalgia patients studied had increased cerebrospinal fluid levels of substance P. Further clarification of the similarities and differences between chronic fatigue syndrome and fibromyalgia may be useful in studies of prognosis and may help define subsets of patients who might benefit from specific therapeutic interventions.

Chronic fatigue syndrome (CFS) is a disease entity of so far unknown etiopathogenesis, without specific markers, that presents with a complex array of symptoms in patients with diverse health histories (see all references cited under this heading in the Bibliography). Fatigue is one of the most prominent features of CFS and one of the most common medical complaints in general. Patients with unexplained chronic pain and/or fatigue have been described for centuries in the medical literature, although the terms used to describe these symptom complexes have changed frequently. Neurasthenia dominated medical thinking at the turn of the century; the term "myalgic encephalomyelitis" was introduced in the United Kingdom in 1957, and, in the mid-1980s, the term "chronic Epstein-Barr virus syndrome" emerged and was then converted to chronic fatigue syndrome and, by some, to "chronic fatigue immune dysfunction syndrome." The currently preferred term, albeit a misnomer, is chronic fatigue syndrome, a name that describes the prominent clinical features of the illness without any attempt to identify the cause but that has the endorsement of the United States Centers for Disease Control and Prevention (CDC) and several professional organizations. Related diseases include fibromyalgia, sick building syndrome, Gulf War syndrome, and multiple chemical sensitivity syndrome. Opinions on CFS range from nondisease via psychiatric disorder to somatic disturbance. Nevertheless, CFS has emerged as a public health concern over the past decade in many countries, and some court rulings have legitimized the diagnosis of CFS in certain societal settings.

The diagnosis of CFS is based on clinical criteria, and it is largely dependent upon ruling out other organic and psychologic causes of fatigue. CFS is defined by primary and secondary criteria, which are, however, largely subjective. CFS includes cases of long-standing (six months or longer) fatigue that are not explained by an existing medical or psychiatric diagnosis and which cause considerable disabilities in professional, social, and/or personal functioning (at least 50 percent reduction in baseline level). Other CFS criteria include: fever, painful adenopathy, muscle weakness, myalgia, headache, migratory arthralgia, neuropsychologic symptoms, and sleep disorder. Although several studies have validated these criteria, much controversy persists and an attempt at formulating new criteria based on laboratory parameters is being attempted. The working case definition of CFS in 1988 was an attempt to establish a uniform basis for the previously heterogeneous approaches to research of this severe and inexplicable state of fatigue. At the same time, researchers wished to narrow down a pathogenetically founded disease entity a priori by specifying precise disease criteria. The case definition has also been used to establish prevalence estimates using physician-based surveillance and random dial telephone surveys. Although the original 1988 definition was revised in 1994, the empirical data gathered in accordance with the CFS definition have failed to confirm the assumption that the disease entity is pathogenetically uniform.

The onset of CFS may be associated with preceding stressful events and multiple other precipitants. A study that divided CFS patients into two groups based on whether onset was sudden or gradual found that the rate of concurrent psychiatric disease was significantly greater in the CFS-gradual group relative to the CFS-sudden group. Although both CFS groups showed a significant reduction in information processing ability relative to controls, impairment in memory was more severe in the CFS-sudden group. Some authors also make a distinction between an acute phase (up to one month after the first consultation), a subacute phase (until six months after the onset of the complaints and disabilities), and a chronic phase (from six months after the onset of the complaints and disabilities) of the disease. CFS evolves toward chronicity in an important number of cases.

Somatic pathogenetic hypotheses for CFS include persisting infections, intoxications, metabolic or immunologic disturbances, nervous system diseases, endocrine pathology, and psychosomatic influences. An infectious illness is not uniformly present at the onset and no single infectious agent has been found. Various components of the central nervous system appear to be involved in CFS, including the hypothalamic pituitary axes, pain-processing pathways, sleep-wake cycle, and autonomic nervous system. Many studies have provided evidence for abnormalities in immunological markers among individuals diagnosed with CFS. Nonetheless, a clear picture has not been achieved in any area of research because of the noticeable variability in the nature and magnitude of the findings reported by different groups. Moreover, little support has been garnered for an association between the laboratory abnormalities and the diverse physical and health status changes in the CFS population. For instance, some authors think that although a subset of CFS patients with immune system activation can be identified, serum markers of inflammation and immune activation are of limited diagnostic usefulness in the evaluation of patients with CFS and chronic fatigue because changes in their values may reflect an intercurrent, transient, common condition, such as an upper respiratory infection, or may be the result of an ongoing illness-associated process. On the other hand, other authors have found that CFS patients can be categorized based on immunological findings or that when patients are classified according to whether the disease started suddenly or gradually, immunological changes are apparent. It is also worth noting that although the degree of overlap between distributions of soluble immune mediators in CFS and controls has fueled criticism on the validity or clinical significance of immune abnormalities in CFS, the latter degree of overlap is not unique to CFS and is also present, for instance, in sepsis syndrome and HIV-1-associated disease, clinical entities where studies of immune abnormalities are providing insight into pathophysiology. The latter statement also applies to nonimmunological parameters in CFS.

Based on the discrepancies described above, some authors argue that the conceptual model of CFS needs to be changed from one determined by a single cause/agent to one in which dysfunction is the end stage of a multifactorial process. A study of author bias in literature citation in CFS reviews revealed that citation of literature is influenced by the authors' disciplines and nationalities, a finding which is compatible with the lack of consensus and integrated efforts among professionals from different disciplines who are working on CFS.

**Cogan I syndrome:** Cogan I syndrome is a rare, inflammatory, systemic disease that is typically characterized by severe audiovestibular dysfunction and various inflammatory eye changes (uveitis, scleritis, keratitis, and episcleritis). In a study of ten patients with Cogan I syndrome, Zierhut et al. (2000) reported other manifestations of this syndrome, including pericarditis associated with arthritis and polyserositis in one patient and fibromyalgia in two patients.

**cognitive-behavioral therapy:** Cognitive-behavioral approaches appear to offer a viable alternative for the management of fibromyalgia and arthritis pain (Bradley and Alberts, 1999; Callahan and Blalock, 1997; Keefe and Caldwell, 1997). In a pilot study of twenty fibromyalgia patients, Singh et al. (1998) showed that a mind-body approach (cognitive-behavioral therapy: eight weekly sessions, two and a half hours each, with three components: an educational component focusing on the mind-body connection, a portion focusing on relaxation response mechanisms, primarily mindfulness meditation techniques, and a qigong movement therapy session) resulted in a significant reduction in pain, fatigue, and sleeplessness; as well as improved function, mood state, and general health. A study by Nicassio et al. (1997) also underscored the value of a ten-week psychoeducational intervention in decreasing the psychological and behavioral effect of fibromyalgia by reducing dysfunctional coping and helplessness. However, in randomized clinical trial comparisons of educational only versus educational-cognitive interventions in 131 fibromyalgia patients, Goossens et al. (1996) and Vlaeyen et al. (1996) found that the addition of a cognitive component to the educational intervention led to significantly higher health care costs (Goossens et al., 2000; Maetzel et al., 1998; Ruof et al., 1999) and no additional improvement in quality of life compared to the educational intervention alone. Some authors suggest the use of mind-body approaches in combination with other interventions (*see* ALTERNATIVE AND COMPLEMENTARY MEDICINE).

**cognitive function:** A study by Grace et al. (1999) on cognitive function reported that thirty fibromyalgia patients studied performed more poorly on tests of immediate and delayed recall and sustained auditory concentration, and their ratings of both their memory abilities and sleep quality were lower than those of the thirty controls. Furthermore, perceived memory deficits of the fibromyalgia subjects were disproportionately greater than their objective deficits. There were also significant correlations between performance on memory and concentration measures and scores on questionnaires of pain severity and trait anxiety. Landro et al. (1997) also reported that, compared to eighteen healthy controls, both twenty-five fibromyalgia patients and twenty-two patients with major depression were significantly impaired on long-term memory tasks requiring effortful processing. However, when the depressive status of the fibromyalgia patients was accounted for, only the subsample with a lifetime major depressive disorder showed memory impairment as compared with the healthy controls.

**collagen:** In a study of thirty-nine fibromyalgia patients, Sprott et al. (1998) found evidence for abnormal collagen metabolism by analyzing urine and serum samples to determine levels of pyridinoline (Pyd) and deoxypyridinoline (Dpyd), which represent products of lysyl oxidase-mediated cross-linking in collagen and are indicators of connective tissue and bone degradation, respectively, and of hydroxypyroline (Hyp), a collagen turnover marker. Based on the findings of significantly decreased urine and serum Pyd/Dpyd ratios and urine Hyp levels in fibromyalgia patients as compared to healthy controls, Sprott et al. (1998) concluded that decreased levels of collagen cross-linking may both contribute to remodeling of the extracellular matrix and collagen deposition around the nerve fibers in fibromyalgia, and underlie the lower pain threshold at the tender points (Malleson, 1998; Sprott and Muller, 1998). The latter results are consistent with the electron microscopic findings of highly ordered cuffs of collagen around the terminal nerve fibers in biopsy tissue from all eight fibromyalgia patients but none of the control skin samples examined by Sprott et al. (1997) in a previous study (*see also* EHLERS-DANLOS SYNDROME).

**coping:** Savelkoul et al. (2000) reported that coping by awaiting/ avoidance in fibromyalgia patients led to less social support and that this decrease in social support negatively influenced subjective well-being. Akkasilpa et al. (2000) found that systemic lupus erythematosus patients with fibromyalgic tender points are less likely to be good "copers," i.e., they display less hardiness. Patient readiness to adopt new beliefs and coping responses to pain may predict response to multidisciplinary or cognitive-behavioral pain treatments that emphasize changes in beliefs and coping behaviors (Jensen et al., 2000). Hellstrom et al. (1999) found that the meaning structures revealed in the patients' ways of describing their experiences of living with fibromyalgia seemed to be partially constituted by their efforts to stand forth as afflicted with a disease, which could be a way to help them to manage the demands that they place upon themselves.

Based on their finding of a relationship between coping strategies and functional disability in fibromyalgia, Martin et al. (1996) suggest that investigators should attempt to identify coping attempts strategies that best reduce patients' psychological distress in the laboratory and then teach patients to use these strategies to reduce distress in their home and work environments. In this regard, Kelley and Clifford (1997) suggest that narrative ethnographic approaches help fibromyalgia patients find both their own strengths and means of coping and their own identities other than as patients. Higher levels of self-efficacy are associated with better outcome (tender point index, disease severity, and pain) and may mediate the effectiveness of rehabilitation-based treatment programs for fibromyalgia in adults and children (Buckelew et al., 1996; Schanberg et al., 1996). In a study of twenty-nine patients, Schanberg et al. (1998) found that family environment and parental pain history may be related to how children cope with fibromyalgia. Behavioral interventions targeting the family may improve the long-term functional status of children with fibromyalgia.

**copper:** A double-blind, with two parallel groups, versus placebo study of forty-eight fibromyalgia patients showed that the use of a pure copper wire bedsheet reduces painful symptomatology at the tender point level and improves sleep quality, with a positive effect on the patients' cenesthesia at awakening (Biasi et al., 1999).

**cortisol:** Hypocortisolism has been reported not only in patients with fibromyalgia but also in those with chronic fatigue syndrome, rheumatoid arthritis, asthma, and post-traumatic stress disorder (Heim et al., 2000). The nature of the underlying mechanisms and the homology of these mechanisms within and across clinical groups remain speculative. Potential mechanisms include dysregulations on several levels of the hypothalamic-pituitary-adrenal axis, genetic vulnerability, previous stress experience, and coping and personality styles (*see also* NEUROENDOCRINOLOGY).

**cryotherapy:** A study by Metzger et al. (2000) of 120 patients, 40.7 percent of whom suffered from primary fibromyalgia, 3.6 percent from secondary fibromyalgia, and the rest from rheumatoid arthritis (17.3 percent), chronic low back pain (16.4 percent), ankylosing spondylitis (10.9 percent), osteoarthritis (9.1 percent), and other autoimmune diseases (1.8 percent) (mean duration of symptoms: four years), concluded that whole-body cold therapy (average 2.5-minute applications, −105°C) generates important short-term effects (decreased pain level for about ninety minutes) and somewhat weaker effects over a four-week treatment period as a whole. Short-term pain reduction facilitates intensive application of physiotherapy and occupational therapy.

 **debrisoquine/sparteine polymorphism:** The scientific literature suggests an association between impaired detoxification and certain diseases, including cancer, Parkinson's disease, fibromyalgia, and chronic fatigue and immune dysfunction syndrome (Liska, 1998). Based on a study of thirty-five fibromyalgia patients, Skeith et al. (1997) found that adverse drug reactions in fibromyalgia patients do not correlate with the poor metabolizer phenotype of the P450IID6 oxidative enzyme. Skeith et al. (1997) also concluded that it is unlikely that altered xenobiotic detoxification attributable to the P450IID6 poor metabolizer phenotype would have a significant role in the development of fibromyalgia.

**dehydroepiandrosterone sulphate:** Dessein et al. (1999) documented hyposecretion of adrenal androgens (dehydroepiandrosterone sulphate, free testosterone) in fifty-seven female fibromyalgia patients. Low serum androgen levels correlated with poor health status, and the decrease in serum androgen levels was more pronounced in obese patients. Longitudinal studies are needed to elucidate whether these are cause and/or effect relationships (*see also* NEUROENDOCRINOLOGY).

**dentistry:** Although mercury exposure from dental amalgam fillings has been proposed as a cause of fibromyalgia and chronic fatigue syndrome, several studies have failed to substantiate this hypothesis (Kotter et al., 1995; Langworth and Stromberg, 1996; Malt et al., 1997). Patients suffering from fibromyalgia can also demonstrate the same clinical features as temporomandibular disorders or myofascial pain. Avon (1996) admonishes that dentists should be aware that certain dental treatments will not be effective in patients suffering from temporal and masseter pain if fibromyalgia has been diagnosed.

**depression:** Wacker (2000) reported comorbidity of depressive disorders and fibromyalgia, and Okifuji et al. (2000) found that although concurrent depressive disorders are prevalent in fibromyalgia (56 percent in a sample of sixty-nine patients) and may be independent of the cardinal features of fibromyalgia, namely, pain severity and hypersensitivity to pressure pain, depressive disorders are related to the cognitive appraisals of the effects of symptoms on daily life and functional activities. Morriss et al. (1999) arrived at a similar conclusion in chronic fatigue syndrome patients in a study where they found that depression is not associated with the reporting of pain, psychophysiological syndromes, and medically unexplained symptoms.

Offenbaecher et al. (1998) reported that of the 27 percent of 304 fibromyalgia patients with depression, 23 percent had a familial history of depression, 46 percent a familial history of fibromyalgia, and 46 percent had been diagnosed with depression in the past. In terms of comorbidity with other psychiatric diagnoses, Kurtze et al. (1998, 1999) found significant effects of anxiety and depression on quality of life, functional disability, and lifestyle among 322 fibromyalgia patients. Anxiety and depression interacted to yield relatively high consumption of coffee and cigarettes among the anxious and depressed subgroup. Meyer-Lindenberg and Gallhofer (1998) recommend that clinical indicators, such as a family history of depressive disorders, circadian disturbances, pronounced loss of appetite or libido, and chronic psychosocial stressors should be assessed and, if present, prompt the initiation of psychiatric evaluation and treatment, including pharmaco- and psychotherapeutic modalities in fibromyalgia patients.

**disability and functional impairment:** Arthritis and other rheumatic conditions (e.g., osteoarthritis, rheumatoid arthritis, gout, fibromyalgia, and other diseases of the joints) are leading causes of disability and are among the most prevalent chronic conditions in the United States, affecting approximately 40 million persons in 1995 and a projected 60 million persons in 2020.

Personal and occupational disability is a serious concern in fibromyalgia (Beger, 1997; Bennett, 1996; Bombardier and Buchwald, 1996; Cohen and Quintner, 1998; Duro, 1997; "Fibromyalgia Syndrome: Feeling More Pain," 1999; Jason et al., 2000; Kaplan et al., 2000; Krapac et al., 1997; Littlejohn, 1998; Pellegrino and Waylonis, 1997; Rocca, 1999; Smith, 1997; Turk et al., 1996; White et al., 1995,

1999; Wolfe, 1996; Wolfe et al., 1997a,b). Gordon (1999) stresses that, despite the presence of disability risk factors, most patients with fibromyalgia maintain a good range of normal daily activities and continue working. Based on a survey of 176 fibromyalgia female patients (50 percent employed, 15 percent full-time, 23 percent not working because of fibromyalgia), Henriksson and Liedberg (2000) recommended early intervention in the work situation by incorporating individual adjustments that allow patients to find a level matching their ability and to continue to work (Henriksson and Burckhardt, 1996). Crook et al. (1998) also recommend that the employer's provision of a "modified job" is important in the prevention of continued disability for workers with musculoskeletal problems.

Several instruments and methods, including the Functional Impact Questionnaire, the Multidimensional Health Questionnaire, the Modified Stanford Health Assessment Questionnaire, the Arthritis Impact Measurement Scales, the Arthritis Self-Efficacy Scales, the Quality of Life Scale, the Medical Outcomes Study Short-Form General Health Survey (SF-36), the Western Ontario MacMaster (WOMAC), the six-minute walk, the Evaluation of Daily Activity Questionnaire (EDAQ), and Multidimensional Pain Inventory, to assess disability and functional limitation in fibromyalgia patients have been tested and are available for different ethnic and linguistic groups (Bakker et al., 1995; Bellamy et al., 1999; Blackmore et al., 1995; Buchwald et al., 1996; Burckhardt and Bjelle, 1996; Buskila and Neumann, 1996; Escalante et al., 1996; Friedman, 1997; Goldenberg et al., 1995; Goossens et al., 1999; Huston, 2000; Kaplan et al., 2000; King et al., 1999; Lousberg et al., 1999; Mannerkorpi and Ekdahl, 1997; Mannerkorpi et al., 1999; Neumann et al., 1999; Neumann, Berzak, et al., 2000; Neumann, Press, et al., 2000; Nordenskiold, 1997; Offenbaecher et al., 2000; Ortiz et al., 1999; Pincus et al., 1999; Wigers, 1996; Wolfe, 1999; Wolfe and Hawtley, 1999; Wolfe and Kong, 1999; Wolfe, 2000; Wolfe et al., 2000).

Despite the availability of the previously mentioned assessment instruments, several authors stress that fibromyalgia is unduly cited as a cause of disability and that it is hard to assess disability in this condition (Keitel, 1999; Kovarsky, 1997; Malterud, 1999; Wolfe and Potter, 1996; Worz, 1999). For instance, Wolfe et al. (1997a,b) found that although most fibromyalgia patients (64 percent of 1,604 surveyed) reported being able to work, there were high rates of self-reported work disability awards. Huber (2000) considers fibromyalgia a psychosomatic disease and points out that a significant proportion of early retirees (at least 30 percent), because of occupational disability, are psychosomatically ill and that an additional large number of retirees suffer from untreatable pain and may have a chronic somatoform pain disorder. Wolfe and Hawley (1999) found that fibromyalgia patients report more medical conditions and report that these conditions are more important to them than do patients with rheumatoid arthritis or osteoarthritis. Van Linthoudt et al. (2000) pointed out that 8 percent of 413 cases seeking insurance compensation in Switzerland were ascribed to fibromyalgia, and admonish that practitioners can contribute to chronicity of rheumatological complaints by perpetuating work interruption for nonmedical reasons. Fibromyalgia also became a major reason for disability pension in Norway. In 1989, more than 7 percent of the new cases had this diagnosis. The parliament (Stortinget) passed controversial amendments to the National Insurance Acts in 1991 and 1995 which restricted the criteria for obtaining a disability pension (Gjesdal and Kristiansen, 1997).

Other authors warn that patients should be made aware that chronic rheumatological complaints do not necessarily result in insurance compensations. A case reported by Mailis et al. (2000) on a family of six all diagnosed with fibromyalgia and who brought the case to court after ten years of significant medical expenses exemplified that compensations are usually used up by legal fees. Moreover, lawyer Karen Capen (1995) and researcher Wolfe (2000) say physicians who provide expert opinion in court should be aware that there are specific requirements regarding their qualifications. In an Alberta, Canada, court case, a judge discounted evidence provided by a rheumatologist who ran a clinic that treated fibromyalgia patients because of his "personal and perhaps financial interest in perpetuating the existence of this condition" (Capen, 1995, p. 207). The judge ruled that "this particular disorder is often found in individuals who will not or cannot cope with everyday stresses of life and convert this inability into acceptable physical symptoms to avoid dealing with reality."

In contrast to the reports mentioned in the previous paragraph, Helfenstein and Feldman (2000) describe their experience with 103 patients referred to a health reference center for workers for the management of repetitive strain injury and work-related arm pain. They found that the patients' illness is far more global than the work-related arm pain that such labeling implies. From the total group, seventy-three fulfilled the American College of Rheumatology criteria for the classification of fibromyalgia syndrome. This means that they were suffering pain above and below the diaphragm, far from the arm pain for which they were referred. These seventy-three patients were clinically and psychologically indistinguishable from 165 patients followed in Helfenstein and Feldman's clinic at the Federal University of Sao Paulo, Rheumatology Division, who also fulfilled these criteria but did not consider their illness to be work related. Some governmental institutions have taken action, and, for instance, the Department of Veterans Affairs of the United States has adopted a rule to add a diagnostic code and evaluation criteria for fibromyalgia to their Schedule for Rating Disabilities (Department of Veterans Affairs, 1999). The intended effect of this rule is to insure that veterans diagnosed with this condition meet uniform criteria and receive consistent evaluations.

A study by Soderberg et al. (1999) highlights the importance of treating people suffering with illness with respect for their human dignity. The findings of the latter study show that being a woman with fibromyalgia means living a life greatly influenced by the illness in various ways: loss of freedom, threat to integrity, and a struggle to achieve relief and understanding. Soderberg et al. (1999) recommend that the care of women with fibromyalgia must empower the women to bring to bear their own resources so that they can manage to live with the illness. Martin et al. (1996) also recommends assessing and improving the patients' coping strategies.

Wolfe et al. (1997a,b) reported that half of 538 fibromyalgia patients studied were dissatisfied with their health, and 59 percent rated their health as fair or poor. In terms of the relevance of fibromyalgia symptomatology, Long et al. (2000) found that although patient satisfaction with health appears to be relatively independent of traditional clinical measures of physical functioning, pain, and disease status among patients with psoriatic arthritis, it was associated with functional class and number of fibromyalgia tender points.

**dizziness:** A study by Rusy et al. (1999) suggests that central (brainstem) and peripheral vestibular (inner ear) mechanisms do not account for the complaints of dizziness in the pediatric patient with fibromyalgia. The common musculoskeletal abnormalities of fibromyalgia may affect their proprioceptive orientation, therefore giving them a sense of imbalance.

 **effort:** Norregaard et al. (1997) found a low degree of effort but near normal physical capacity in a study of 181 female fibromyalgia patients. Fibromyalgia patients exhibited a significant reduction in voluntary muscle strength of the knee and elbow, and flexors and extensors in the order of 20 to 30 percent. However, the coefficient of variation was higher among patients, thus indicating lower effort. Moreover, unlike work status, degree of effort or physical capacity did not correlate to psychometric scores.

**Ehlers-Danlos syndrome:** Fibromalgia may be concurrent with Ehlers-Danlos syndrome (Miller et al., 1997), a disease characterized by a genetic defect in collagen synthesis (*see* COLLAGEN).

**eosinophilia-myalgia syndrome:** The eosinophilia-myalgia syndrome (EMS), caused by intake of contaminated L-tryptophan, resembles fibromyalgia in its clinical presentation (Barth et al., 1999; Hudson et al., 1996). In one study, the similar incidence (81 percent) of myalgia and arthralgia and the presence of antibodies directed against serotonin, gangliosides, and phospholipids in both chronic EMS and fibromyalgia patients, as well as the predominant production of type 2 cytokines in vitro after stimulation with different L-tryptophan preparations of peripheral blood mononuclear cells from fibromyalgia patients, led Barth et al. (1999) to postulate that EMS may have developed in patients suffering primarily from fibromyalgia as an allergic reaction toward a more immunogenic L-tryptophan preparation. Nonetheless, Taylor et al. (1996) point out that four variables, namely extremity edema, leukocyte count greater than 12.5 × $10^9$/L, dyspnea, and absence of arthralgias, differentiate EMS from other common myalgia syndromes (sensitivity of 95.6 percent, a specificity of 96.9 percent, and positive and negative predictive values of 93.5 and 97.9 percent, respectively).

**epidemiology:** In 1995, an estimated 15 percent (40 million) of Americans had some form of musculoskeletal pain disorder, including fibromyalgia, and, by the year 2020, an estimated 18.2 percent (59.4 million) will be affected (Lawrence et al., 1998). Pain syndromes can be divided anatomically into those that cause generalized pain, such as fibromyalgia syndrome and myofascial pain syndromes, and those that are confined to one regional anatomical area. The latter group comprise those of the neck, shoulder, elbow, wrist/hand, hip, knee, and ankle/foot (Linaker et al., 1999). Fibromyalgia can also be secondary to other rheumatologic disorders (Karaaslan et al., 1999).

It is estimated that fibromyalgia affects up to 6 million patients worldwide (Gordon and Morrison, 1998; Smith, 1998). The prevalence of fibromyalgia in the United States general population was found to be 2 percent, and increases with age (Goldenberg, 1996). Extrapolation of a survey of 4,027 general practitioners by Bazelmans et al. (1997) indicates that in 1997 there were at least 24,000 primary fibromyalgia patients in the Netherlands. A population survey of 2,498 females living in South Norway yielded a calculated annual incidence of fibromyalgia of 583 per 100,000 (Forseth, 1997; Forseth et al., 1997). Major problems associated with interpreting and comparing epidemiologic studies on pain syndromes in adults and children include the diversity of classification criteria and selection bias (Gare, 1996). The prevalence of fibromyalgia in a study of 548 schoolchildren by Clark et al. (1998) was 1.2 percent, a figure that is fivefold lower than previously reported. This variance may be due to: (1) racial and sociocultural differences between populations; and (2) differences in methodological approach. However, Sardini et al. (1996) found the same incidence of fibromyalgia of 1.2 percent in students of the schools of Castiglione delle Stiviere (Mantova, Italy).

Case definitions and overlap between different syndromes affect the results of the different epidemiological studies. For example, of 32 individuals with chronic fatigue syndrome identified in a random sample of 18,675 Chicago residents, 40.6 percent met criteria for multiple chemical sensitivity and 15.6 percent met criteria for fibromyalgia (Jason et al., 2000). Referral practices and primary care physicians' perceptions of fibromyalgia (Bellamy et al., 1998) also affect epidemiological estimates. For instance, Gran and Nordvag (2000) found that the annual incidence of referrals of new patients to a rheumatology clinic was 423 per 100,000. The main cause of referral was diagnosis, and more than half of the diagnoses suggested were changed at the visit. Few of the referred patients had severe disease.

In a study of 100 confirmed fibromyalgia cases, 76 widespread pain controls, and 135 general controls in a random community survey of 3,395 noninstitutionalized adults living in London, Ontario, White, Harth, et al., (1999), and White et al., (1999a-c) found that adults who meet the American College of Rheumatology definition of fibromyalgia appear to have four distinct features compared to those with chronic widespread pain who do not meet criteria, namely pain severity, severe fatigue lasting twenty-four hours after minimal activity, weakness, and self-reported swelling of neck glands. In a different report from the same study, White et al. (1999c) reported that being female, middle-aged, of less education, lower household income, being divorced, and being disabled are associated with increased odds of having fibromyalgia. White et al. (1999b) also determined that fibromyalgia has a major effect on direct health care costs. The latter is particularly relevant because fibromyalgia is prevalent among lower income people. In a study of 1,997 Pakistani adults distributed evenly between poor rural and poor urban communities and relatively affluent urban people, Farooqi and Gibson (1998) found that there was significantly more soft tissue rheumatism and back pain in the rural population compared with those in the city. Fibromyalgia was almost completely absent from the urban affluent, but osteoarthritis of the knee was significantly more common in this community, perhaps due to relative obesity. In contrast with the latter results, no chronic widespread pain was identified in a survey of Pima indians, a finding that suggests that this population has different pain perception or different patterns of risk factors for these disorders (Jacobsson et al., 1996).

**Epstein-Barr virus:** Rheumatologic complications of infections with herpes viruses, such as the Epstein-Barr virus, need to be included in the differential for the diagnosis of fibromyalgia (McCarty and Csuka, 1998).

*Erb* **gene:** Lowe et al. (1997) have proposed the hypothesis that in euthyroid fibromyalgia a mutant c-*erbA beta 1* gene (or alternately, the c-*erbA alpha 1* gene) results in low-affinity thyroid hormone receptors that prevent normal thyroid hormone regulation of transcription. As in hypothyroidism, this would cause a shift toward alpha-adrenergic dominance and increases in both cyclic adenosine 3'-5'-phosphate phosphodiesterase and inhibitory G proteins. The result would be tissue-specific hypothyroid-like symptoms despite normal circulating thyroid hormone levels.

**ergonomics:** Working daily for a long time with a standard microscope causes back pain, soft tissue rheumatism or fibromyalgia, or tension headache in up to 80 percent of microscopists. These complaints may be prevented by an ergonomic design of the microscope workstation, leading to a beneficial and significant reduction of electromyographical activity in the most strained muscle groups, as shown by surface electromyographic recordings (Kreczy et al., 1999; Van Houdenhove and Neerinckx, 1999).

**erythrocyte sedimentation rate:** In a study of 711 patients referred to rheumatology clinics, Suarez-Almazor et al. (1998) found that primary care physicians frequently requested erythrocyte sedimentation rate (ESR) (29 percent) in patients with fatigue and diffuse musculoskeletal pain. The majority of test results were negative, which caused low predictive values for positive ESR tests (35 percent for connective tissue disease, 17 percent for rheumatoid arthritis, and 3 percent for systemic lupus erythematosus). Suarez-Almazor et al. (1998) admonished that a decrease in inappropriate ESR test ordering could be achieved by emphasizing that fatigue and diffuse musculoskeletal pain are not indicative of connective tissue disease in the absence of other features such as joint swelling, typical rash, or organ involvement.

**exercise:** Exercise programs alone or in combination with other interventions have proven useful in the treatment of fibromyalgia (Buckelew et al., 1998; Deuster, 1996; Dominick et al., 1999; Wigers et al., 1996). The type, duration, and intensity of the exercise program deserves special consideration. Training has shown little benefit as regards pain but has improved the physical fitness of the patients. Since pain may be exacerbated by physical activity, many patients become physically inactive, with possible development of reduced physical fitness. In the long run, fibromyalgia patients who exercise report fewer symptoms than sedentary patients do. Thus, exercise should be aimed at preventing physical inactivity and improving the patients' physical fitness (Mengshoel, 1996).

A study of fifty-eight fibromyalgia patients by Mannerkorpi et al. (2000) concluded that six months of exercises in a temperate pool combined with a six-session education program improve physical function, grip strength, pain severity, social functioning, psychological distress, and quality of life. Gowans et al. (1999) found similar efficacy for a six-week exercise and educational program tested on forty-one subjects. Meiworm et al. (2000) reported a positive effect for twelve weeks of aerobic endurance exercise (jogging, walking, cycling, or swimming) on pain parameters, cardiovascular status, fitness, and well-being of twenty-seven fibromyalgia patients compared to sedentary patient controls. Ramsay et al. (2000) found that although there was no improvement in pain in a study of seventy-four fibromyalgia patients following either a supervised twelve-week aerobic exercise class or unsupervised home aerobic exercises, there was some significant benefit in psychological well-being in the exercise class group and perhaps a slowing of functional deterioration. Based on a limited study, Meyer and Lemley (2000) suggest that individuals with fibromyalgia can adhere to low-intensity walking programs two to three times per week, possibly reducing fibromyalgia impact on daily activities. Self-help programs that include stretching exercises are also beneficial (Han, 1998).

A study of thirty-eight fibromyalgia patients by Martin et al. (1996) showed that an exercise program that included aerobic, flexibility, and strengthening elements had no adverse effects and was effective in the short term. Normal muscle metabolism during exercise and no muscle damage after physical activity have been reported in fibromyalgia patients (Mengshoel et al., 1995; Mengshoel, 1996). However, no rise in blood noradrenaline concentration during exercise was found in fibromyalgia patients.

**F**atigue: A study of 1,488 patients by Wolfe et al. (1996) documented that fatigue is common across all rheumatic diseases, is associated with all measures of distress, and is a predictor of work dysfunction and overall health status. The correlates of fatigue (pain, sleep disturbances, and disability) are generally similar across fibromyalgia, rheumatoid arthritis, and osteoarthritis. However, in a review of 425 medical charts, Ward et al. (1996) found that the workup for chronic fatigue is often incomplete or lacks documentation. This oversight is likely due to the problem that focus is not being directed at the chronic fatigue complaints. Also complicating the evaluation process are the multiple associated disorders, the prevalence of the complaint, and cost/benefit issues facing the primary care physician (Groopman, 1998; Llewelyn, 1996; Ream and Richardson, 1996; Shapiro, 1998; Tiesinga et al., 1996; White, 1997). Fatigue is a complex, multicausal, multidimensional, nonspecific, and subjective phenomenon for which no single definition is widely accepted. The condition of fatigue requires adequate assessment, innovative planning and interventions, and patient-centered evaluations by health care professionals. Fatigue, whether acute or chronic, needs to be recognized as a true and valid condition for treatment to be successful. Chronic fatigue and acute fatigue can be quite different conditions, requiring different approaches. Miller et al. (1996) reported that neither poor motivation, reflex pain inhibition, nor muscle contractile failure are important in the pathogenesis of fatigue in fibromyalgia patients. However, the subjective response to exercise is commonly excessive.

**fibromyalgia:** Fibromyalgia is a form of nonarticular, or soft tissue, rheumatism characterized by spontaneous widespread musculoskeletal aching, tenderness on palpation with multiple tender points (at least eleven out of eighteen in defined locations) (hyperalgesia), decreased pain threshold (allodynia), fatigue, poor sleep, mood disturbances, and other systemic symptoms (Ang and Wilke, 1999; Bennett, 1998; Briggs, 1997; Celiker et al., 1997; Clauw, 1995; Coward, 1999; "Fibromyalgia," 2000; "Fibromyalgia Syndrome," 1997; Fordyce, 2000; Gerster, 1999; Gordon and Morrison, 1998; Hadler, 1996a,b; Healey, 1996; Krsnich-Shriwise, 1997; Leslie, 1999; Lilleaas, 1997; Littlejohn, 1996; MacFarlane et al., 1996; Mailis, 1996; Nishikai, 1999; Parziale and Chen, 1996; Pasero, 1998; Proceedings of the International Fibromyalgia Conference, 1998; Rankin, 1999; Raspe and Croft, 1995; Reiffenberger and Amundson, 1996; Reveille, 1997; Reynolds, 1996; Romano, 1996; Siegmeth, 1999; Simms, 1996; Slavkin, 1997; Tabeeva et al., 2000; Unger, 1996; Van Santen-Hoeufft, 1996; Wallace, 1999; Wallace et al., 1999; Winfield, 1997; Wootton, 2000; Xie and Ye, 1997). The concept and diagnosis of fibromyalgia became popular, especially in North America, in the 1970s. It is noticeable that there does not appear to be an early case report, as there is, for instance, for gout, rheumatoid arthritis, or certain vasculitides. Operational definitions and classification criteria were given in 1990, with the endorsement of the American College of Rheumatology and are now the most widely used. Although nearly all rheumatologists now accept fibromyalgia as a distinct diagnostic entity, and it is also recognized by the World Health Organization, the validity of fibromyalgia as a distinct clinical entity has been challenged for several reasons: the subjective nature of chronic pain; the subjectivity of the tender point examination; the failure to agree on the importance and biological nature of tenderness itself; the lack of a gold standard laboratory test; the absence of a clear pathogenic mechanism; the use of a syndromic description without a unifying concept; the relative nature of the pain-distress relationship in the rheumatology clinic; the apparently continuous relationship between tender points and somatic distress across a variety of clinical disorders; the failure to distinguish a clinical feature from a disease process; legal defenses of insurance carriers motivated by economic concerns; psychiatric dogma; uninformed posturing; suspicion of malingering; ignorance of nociceptive physiology; and, occasionally, honest misunderstanding (Buskila et al., 1997; Cathebras et al., 1998; Cathebras, 2000; Cohen, 1999; Finestone, 1997; Fitzcharles, 1999; Gamaz-Nava et al., 1998; Goldenberg, 1999; Gordon, 1997; Hadler, 1996a,b, 1997a,b; Hamilton, 1998; Handler, 1998; Hantzschel and Boche, 1999; Helliwell, 1995; Hellstrom, 1995; Hilden, 1996; Holoweiko, 1996; Hudson, 1998; Hunt et al., 1998; Hyams, 1998; Jones, 1996; Kaden and Bubenzer, 1999; Katz et al., 1997; Kissel and Mahnig, 1998; Laser, 1998; Leonhardt, 2000; Lindberg and Lindberg, 2000; Makela, 1999; Marlowe, 1998; Matsumoto, 1999; Neeck, 1998; Neerinckx et al., 2000; Peloso, 1998; Quintner and Cohen, 1997, 1999; Raspe, 1996; Rau and Russell, 2000; Rekola et al., 1997; Romano, 1998; Russell, 1999; Safran, 1998; Shojania, 2000; Smith MD, 1998; Smith WA, 1998; Solomon and Liang, 1997; Thorson, 1998; Wessely and Hotopf, 1999; White and Harth, 1998; Wigley, 1999; Wilke, 1996a,b; Wolfe, 1997; Wolfe et al., 1997). In the United States, fibromyalgia is the third or fourth most common reason for rheumatology referral (Celiker et al., 1997; Gamez-Nava et al., 1998; Wallace, 1997) and several Web sites are dedicated to this condition (Armstrong, 2000; Jahn and Klenke, 1999). Fibromyalgia is predominant in middle-aged women but has also been reported in men, elderly individuals, and in the pediatric population (Borenstein, 1996; Buskila, 1999; Cathebras et al., 1998; Holland and Gonzalez, 1998).

According to the American College of Rheumatology, the diagnosis of fibromyalgia is based on criteria consisting entirely of clinical signs and symptoms (Alarcon, 1997; Barth, 1997; Bassetti, 1996; Brown, 1997; Garfin, 1995; Hart, 1998; Jacobsen, 2000; Kavanaugh, 1996; Kjaergaard, 1998; Maier, 1998; Pongratz and Sievers, 2000; Reinhold-Keller, 1997; "Unraveling a Mysterious Cause of Pain," 1998; Weber, 1998; Xie and Ye, 1997; Zborovskii and Babaeva, 1998). The American College of Rheumatology criteria, established in 1990, provide the primary care provider with definitive subjective and objective findings that have shown to be 88 percent accurate in their ability to diagnose patients with the syndrome (Smith MD, 1998; Smith WA, 1998). In the majority of fibromyalgia patients generalized pain is preceded by localized or regional pain, usually in the musculoskeletal system. In many fibromyalgia patients there are findings compatible with tissue injury pain, with pain mechanisms involving both the primary afferent neuron and the nociceptive system in the central nervous system (Henriksson, 1999; Olin and Lidbeck, 1996). The distinction between fibromyalgia (tender points) and myofascial pain syndrome (trigger points) is essential (Klineberg et al., 1998; Uppgaard, 2000) (*see* TENDER POINT PATHOPHYSIOLOGY; *see also* TRIGGER POINTS). Also, macrophagic myofasciitis, a recently identified inflammatory myopathy that can be detected by deltoid muscle biopsy and is manifested mainly in the lower limbs, can be differentiated from fibromyalgia and sarcoidosis by gallium-67 scintigraphy (Cherin et al., 2000). Fitzcharles and Esdaile (1997) reported that eleven women with spondyloarthritis had been incorrectly diagnosed as having fibromyalgia. Internal and neurological disorders as a primary cause of fibromyalgia have to be excluded (Olin and Lidbeck, 1996).

The etiology and pathogenesis of fibromyalgia still remain uncertain, and some reports suggest a genetic component (Bennett, 1998; Gelfand, 1998; Kelly, 1997; Kenner, 1998; Monroe, 1998; Shelkovnikov and Krivoruchko, 1997). Fibromyalgia symptoms last, on average, at least fifteen years after illness onset (de Jesus, 2000; Kennedy and Felson, 1996). However, most patients experience some improvement in symptoms before that time (Kennedy and Felson, 1996). Patients with fibromyalgia report greater difficulty in performing activities of daily living as well as increased pain, fatigue, and weakness compared with healthy controls (Bennett, 1998; Celiker et al., 1997; Hadler, 1996a,b; Kennedy and Felson, 1996; MacFarlane et al., 1996; Slavkin, 1997). Associated disorders are restless leg syndrome, irritable bowel syndrome, irritable bladder syndrome, interstitial cystitis, headaches, ocular and vestibular complaints, cognitive dysfunction, cold intolerance, multiple sensitivities, and dizziness (Asencio-Marchante and Terriza-Garcia, 1998; Bennett, 1998; Maurizio and Rogers, 1997; Siegmeth, 1999). Some muscle abnormalities have been reported (Park et al., 1998); the myopathological patterns in fibromyalgia are nonspecific: type II fiber atrophy, an increase of lipid droplets, a slight proliferation of mitochondria, and a slightly elevated incidence of ragged red fibers (Pongratz and Sievers, 2000). However, most studies agree on an absence of inflammatory or structural musculoskeletal abnormalities (Matsumoto, 1999), and, therefore, the original term "fibrositis" was replaced with fibromyalgia (Simms, 1998).

There is clinical, and in many cases demographic, overlap between fibromyalgia, chronic fatigue syndrome, Persian Gulf War syndrome, silicone implant-associated syndrome, sick building syndrome, multiple chemical sensitivity, and syndromes including neurally mediated hypotension, abnormalities of the growth hormone-insulin-like growth factor-1 axis, chemical intolerance, altered functioning of the stress-response system, and the presence of autoantibodies (Baschetti, 1999; Bazelmans et al., 1997; Bennett, 1998; Buchwald, 1996; Buskila, 1999, 2000; Chambers, 1997; Csef, 1999; Goldenberg, 1997; Granzow, 1999; Hoffmann et al., 1996; Kelly, 1997; Kenner, 1998; Klimas, 1998; Pocinki, 1997; Robertson, 1999; Sabal, 1997; Slavkin, 1997; Vree, 1997; Wallace, 1997; Wessely and Hotopf, 1999). However, there are differences among the latter syndromes (Matsumoto, 1999). Fibromyalgia may also be affected by psychosocial, cultural, psychological, and environmental factors (Affleck et al., 1998; Ben-Zion et al., 1996; Cathebras, 1997; Hadler, 1996a,b; Hausotter, 1998; Kissel and Mahnig, 1998; Kuhn, 2000; Kurtze et al., 1998; Reid et al., 1997; Schaefer, 1997; Schuck et al., 1997; Turk et al., 1996). On the other hand, fibromyalgia may complicate other syndromes (Kelemen and Muller, 1998; Potter, 1997), as is the case in some patients with hyperlaxity syndromes, such as benign joint hypermobility syndrome (Grahame, 2000).

Fibromyalgia patients journey along a continuum from experiencing symptoms, through seeking a diagnosis, to coping with the illness. Experiencing symptoms usually entails pain, a precipitating event, associated symptoms, and modulating factors. Seeking a diagnosis is associated with frustration and social isolation. Confirmation of diagnosis brings relief but anxiety about the future. After diagnosis, several steps lead to creation of adaptive coping strategies (Mannekorpi et al., 1999; Raymond and Brown, 2000; Thorson, 1999). Treatment of patients with fibromyalgia and CFS continues to be of limited success, although the role of multidisciplinary group intervention appears promising (Bennett, 1998; Celiker et al., 1997; Goldenberg, 1996, 1997; Hadler, 1996a,b; MacFarlane et al., 1996; Slavkin, 1997) and several strategies have proven useful (Keitel, 1997; Maidannik, 1996; Moldofsky et al., 1996; Reiffenberger and Amundson, 1996; Scharf et al., 1998; Stoll, 2000; Wilke, 1996a,b). The conventional medical model fails to address the complex experience of fibromyalgia, and adopting a patient-centered approach is important for helping patients cope with this disease (Cunningham, 1996; Fitzcharles, 1999; Hellstrom et al., 1998; Leslie, 1999; Raymond and Brown, 2000; Romano, 1999; Smith MD, 1998; Smith WA, 1998).

**fitness:** Although regular physical activity is associated with important physical and mental health benefits, an estimated 53 million U.S. adults are inactive during their leisure time—the period most amenable to efforts to increase physical activity. The presence of chronic conditions, especially those associated with disabilities, may reduce levels of leisure time physical activity, and a government report documented a decreased leisure-time physical activity prevalence among persons with arthritis and other rheumatic conditions, such as fibromyalgia ("Prevalence of Leisure-Time Physical Activity," 1997).

Nielens et al. (2000) found that cardiorespiratory fitness, as expressed by a submaximal work capacity index, seems normal, despite increased perceived exertion scores, in thirty female fibromyalgia patients compared with sixty-seven age- and sex-matched healthy individuals. However, Natvig et al. (1998) reported that fibromyalgia patients had higher physical leisure activity levels, but lower physical fitness than the control women in a population survey. The difference in physical leisure activity persisted even after controlling for a series of possible confounders, including employment status and workload. Fitness should therefore be objectively assessed before recommending interventions involving physical activity in fibromyalgia patients.

**functional somatic syndromes:** Barsky and Borus (1999), among other authors (Ford, 1997; Masi, 1998; Robbins et al., 1997; Walker et al., 1997), have applied the term functional somatic syndromes to several related syndromes characterized more by symptoms, suffering, and disability than by consistently demonstrable tissue abnormality. These syndromes include multiple chemical sensitivity, sick building syndrome, repetition stress injury, the side effects of silicone breast implants, Gulf War syndrome, chronic whiplash, chronic fatigue syndrome, irritable bowel syndrome, and fibromyalgia. Barsky and Borus (1999) purport that although discrete pathophysiologic causes may ultimately be found in some patients with functional somatic syndromes, the suffering of these patients is exacerbated by a self-perpetuating, self-validating cycle in which common, endemic, somatic symptoms are incorrectly attributed to serious abnormality, reinforcing the patient's belief that he or she has a serious disease. Ford (1997) considers these syndromes a "fashionable" way to hide the diagnosis of hysteria.

**Gamma-hydroxybutyrate:** A preliminary study found that gamma-hydroxybutyrate administered in divided doses at night in eleven fibromyalgia patients resulted in significant improvement in both fatigue and pain, with an increase in slow-wave sleep and a decrease in the severity of the alpha anomaly (Russell, 1999; Scharf et al., 1998).

**gender:** The heterogeneous group of diseases that causes chronic arthralgia and arthritis is the most common cause of activity limitation and disability among middle aged and older women (Holtedahl, 1999; Stormorken and Brosstad, 1999). For reasons that remain poorly understood, this group of diseases affects women substantially more frequently than men (Belilos and Carsons, 1998; Forseth et al., 1999; Meisler, 1999). In particular, the prevalence rates of the most common causes of arthralgia and arthritis, osteoarthritis and rheumatoid arthritis, and the prevalence rates of less common diseases that cause arthralgia, including systemic lupus erythematosus, systemic sclerosis, and fibromyalgia, are between two and ten times higher in women (Buckwalter and Lappin, 2000; Burckhardt and Bjelle, 1996). Forseth et al. (1997) estimated an annual incidence of fibromyalgia in women of 583 per 100,000. Because many women with these conditions seek medical care from orthopaedists, orthopaedic residency education and continuing medical education should place emphasis on early diagnosis and nonoperative treatment of patients with arthralgia and arthritis and, when appropriate, early referral to rheumatologists (Schaefer, 1997).

A study by Buskila et al. (2000), comparing forty men and forty women with fibromyalgia, concluded that although fibromyalgia is uncommon in men, its health outcome is worse than in women (more severe symptoms, decreased physical function, and lower quality of life in men despite similar mean tender point counts). In contrast to the latter study, Yunus et al. (2000), in a comparative study of sixty-seven men and 469 women with fibromyalgia, found that male fibromyalgia patients had fewer symptoms and fewer tender points, and less common "hurt all over" complaints, fatigue, morning fatigue, and irritable bowel syndrome, compared with female patients. Further studies of gender comparisons are needed.

**genetics:** A familial inheritance of fibromyalgia is suggested by the report by Buskila and Neumann (1997), who found that relatives of fibromyalgia patients have a higher prevalence (26 percent: 14 percent in male relatives and 41 percent in female relatives) of fibromyalgia and suffer more nonarticular point tenderness than the general population. Moreover, Buskila et al. (1996) also reported a high prevalence (28 percent) of fibromyalgia among offspring of fibromyalgic mothers. Because psychological and familial factors were not different in children with and without fibromyalgia, the high familial occurrence of this syndrome may be attributable to genetic factors. In terms of possible genes involved, the serotonin transporter promoter gene seems to be associated with neurotic anxiety and fibromyalgia (Ackenheil, 1998) (*see also* SEROTONIN RECEPTOR GENE). Several studies by Yunus (1998) and Yunus et al. (1999) have suggested the existence of a possible gene for fibromyalgia that is linked with the human leukocyte antigen (HLA) region (Buskila, 2000). In contrast to the latter findings in fibromyalgia, myofascial temporomandibular disorder does not run in families (Buskila, 2000). Klein and Berg (1995) also found a higher frequency of an autoantibody pattern, characteristically found among fibromyalgia patients and consisting of antiganglioside, antiphospholipid, and antiserotonin antibodies, among relatives of fibromyalgia patients.

**glucocorticoid:** Ernberg et al. (1997) reported that patients with fibromyalgia and those with localized myalgia of the masseter muscle show a similar positive response (decreased pain to palpation) to local glucocorticoid treatment, an observation that points to a possible common pathophysiology in both disorders.

**growth hormone:** The various components of the growth hormone (GH)-insulin-like growth factor (IGF-I) axis and their binding proteins have many peripheral effects, mainly on bone, growth, activation of main cellular functions, energy metabolism, and protein anabolism. They contribute to adapting an individual to circumstances of life and illness (Schlienger and Goichot, 1998). It has been suggested that growth hormone deficiency may be a pathogenic factor in fibromyalgia, and decreased serum levels of IGF-I, a surrogate marker for low growth hormone secretion, are common in fibromyalgia patients (Bennett, 1998; Berwaerts et al., 1998; Leal-Cerro et al., 1999). Growth hormone deficiency is characterized by diminished energy, dysphoria, impaired cognition, poor general health, reduced exercise capacity, muscle weakness, and cold intolerance. However, Dinser et al. (2000) found that in only one of fifty-six subjects tested did growth hormone levels remain below 3 ng/mL after hypoglycemia and additional arginine stimulation, an observation that satisfies the criteria for adult growth hormone deficiency. Dinser et al. (2000) and Bennett (1998) also observed an impaired reactivity of the somatotropic axis in one-third of fibromyalgia patients, in keeping with other studies that have found a functional alteration of the hypothalamus. For instance, Leal-Cerro et al. (1999) found that fibromyalgia patients exhibit a marked decrease in spontaneous growth hormone secretion, but normal pituitary responsiveness to exogenously administered growth hormone releasing hormone. Defective growth hormone secretion in fibromyalgia patients appears to be due to increased somatostatin tone in the hypothalamus, which in turn may be secondary to upregulation of beta-adrenergic receptors in the hypothalamus (Bennett, 1998; Bennett et al., 1998). Although some preliminary studies have shown that treatment of growth hormone-deficient fibromyalgia patients with recombinant growth hormone (daily for nine months) improves several clinical features, including the tender point count, large double-blind, placebo-controlled clinical trials are needed (Bagge et al., 1998; Bennett, 1998; Bennett et al., 1998; Schlienger and Goichot, 1998).

**gynecology:** A strong association between musculoskeletal disorders and gynecological disease was found by Wadsworth et al. (1995) and Ostensen and Schei (1997). In the latter study, differences between healthy women and women reporting pelvic joint syndrome, fibromyalgia, whiplash, or arthritis were significant in terms of bleeding disorders, chronic pelvic pain, and inflammatory pelvic disease. ter Borg et al. (1999) have also reported a high frequency of hysterectomies among fibromyalgia patients.

**hair electrolytes:** Some patients with fibromyalgia were observed to have high hair calcium and magnesium levels compared with healthy subjects; in these patients supplementing calcium with magnesium reduces the number of tender points detected by digital palpation (Ng, 1999).

**headache:** According to a model presented based on the data from Bendtsen (2000), the main problem in chronic tension-type headaches, myofascial pain syndromes, and fibromyalgia is central sensitization at the level of the spinal dorsal horn/trigeminal nucleus due to prolonged nociceptive inputs from pericranial myofascial tissues. The increased nociceptive input to supraspinal structures may in turn result in supraspinal sensitization. The central neuroplastic changes may affect the regulation of peripheral mechanisms and thereby lead to, for example, increased pericranial muscle activity or release of neurotransmitters in the myofascial tissues. By such mechanisms, the central sensitization may be maintained even after the initial eliciting factors have been normalized, resulting in the conversion of episodic into chronic tension-type headaches, or of episodic pain into the chronic pain of fibromyalgia (Bendtsen, 2000). Okifuji et al. (1999) reported that extensive dysregulation in pain modulation is important for a substantial minority of recurrent headache patients (twenty-eight out of seventy studied), who seem to be quite similar to fibromyalgia patients (presence of widespread tender point pain suggesting generalized hyperalgesia). Defects in serotonergic analgesia and hyperalgesic states are proposed as features common to headache and fibromyalgia (Nicolodi and Sicuteri, 1996; Nicolodi et al., 1998). The benefit to both migraine and fibromyalgia from inhibiting ionotropic N-methyl-D-aspartate receptor activity implies that redundant hyperalgesia-related neuroplastic changes are crucial for severe or chronic migraine and primary fibromyalgia. In fact, there is a high prevalence of migraine in the population of fibromyalgia sufferers, and migraine may represent a risk factor for fibromyalgia (Nicolodi and Sicuteri, 1996; Nicolodi et al., 1998).

Because of the similarities mentioned, chronic tension-type headache, premenstrual headache, and migraines are in the differential of the fibromyalgia diagnosis. Fox and Davis (1998) documented chronobiological features that may assist in the differential diagnosis of migraine: Migraine attacks start more frequently between 4 a.m. and 9 a.m. and within the first few days after onset of menses; this migraine periodicity is strongest among women not using oral contraceptives. Seasonal periodicity, if any, is clearly weaker than circadian or menstrual. Paiva et al. (1995) documented that polysomnography was useful in the diagnosis of patients presenting with morning and nocturnal headaches: thirteen out of fifteen patients had their diagnosis changed from one of the headache entities (cluster, chronic paroxysmal hemicrania, migraine, tension, combined headache, and chronic substance abuse headache) to periodic movements of sleep, fibromyalgia syndrome, and obstructive sleep apnea. In terms of differential response to treatment, Stone and Wharton (1997) reported that the application of a unique physical therapy device combining transcutaneous electrical nerve stimulation, traction, massage, vibration, and acupressure applied to the forehead, posterior cervical spine, and scapula yielded improvement for neck pain and headache patients, but fibromyalgia trigger points were unaffected. In contrast to patients with chronic tension-type headaches, Schepelmann et al. (1998) found no changes of the second suppressive period of the exteroceptive suppression of the temporalis muscle activity in fibromyalgia patients.

**hearing:** Although central nervous system dysfunction frequently occurs in fibromyalgia patients, proprioceptive disturbances might also explain some of the abnormalities observed. Rosenhall et al.

(1996) reported that 72 percent of 168 fibromyalgia patients studied suffered from vertigo/dizzines, 15 percent were afflicted with sensorineural hearing loss, 30 percent had evidence of brainstem dysfunction, 28 percent had abnormal saccades and 58 percent had pathological smooth pursuit eye movements in oculomotor studies, and 45 percent had a pathological electronystagmography. On the other hand, Heller et al. (1998) reported that twenty-eight of eighty patients with sudden deafness and progressive hearing losses (approximately half of whom had phospholipid antibodies that can cause venous or arterial vasculopathies, or serotonin and ganglioside antibodies) displayed symptoms typical for fibromyalgia and chronic fatigue disorders, including fatigue, myalgia, arthralgia, depressions, sicca symptoms, and diarrhea. Klein and Berg (1995) described a higher frequency of the latter autoantibody pattern among relatives of fibromyalgia patients. Heller et al. (1998) recommend questioning patients suffering from inner ear disorders for symptoms typical for fibromyalgia or chronic fatigue, since these diseases are often closely related to inner ear disorders. If symptoms are present, antibodies should be tested against phospholipids, serotonin, and gangliosides.

Dohrenbusch et al. (1997) found reduced unpleasantness thresholds for all audiometric frequencies and an asymptomatic hearing loss for higher frequencies among thirty fibromyalgia patients compared to thirty-six matched controls. The hearing loss correlated significantly with experience of noise at the place of work, which was also elevated in the fibromyalgia group. Generalized pain had a high impact on the interaction between threshold of unpleasantness and daily noise experience. Dohrenbusch et al. (1997) interpreted the differences in thresholds of hearing and of unpleasantness in patients with fibromyalgia as a form of either preconscious or conscious acts to protect against disturbing stimulation. The latter results support the notion of a generalized disturbance of perceptual thresholds in patients with fibromyalgia not restricted to the perception of pain (Kroner-Herwig, 1997).

**hepatitis C:** Hepatitis C virus (HCV) is both a hepatotropic and a lymphotropic virus; because of this latter biological peculiarity, HCV may trigger a constellation of autoimmune-lymphoproliferative disorders. Rheumatologic complications of HCV infection are common and include mixed cryoglobinemia, vasculitis, sicca symptoms, myalgia, arthritis, carpal tunnel syndrome, tenosynovitis, and fibromyalgia (Barkhuizen and Bennett, 1997; Buskila, 2000; Ferri and Zignego, 2000; Jendro et al., 1997; Killenberg, 2000; Lovy et al., 1996; Rivera et al., 1997). However, rheumatic complications are not associated with liver disease severity, subjects' gender, presence of autoantibodies (cryoglobulins, rheumatoid factor, antinuclear antibodies, antismooth muscle antibodies, antiphospholipid antibodies, and antithyroid antibodies) or response to treatment with interferon-alpha (Buskila et al., 1998; Buskila, 2000; Jendro et al., 1997; Rivera et al., 1997). The identification of HCV infection in rheumatic patients is important to minimize the risk of aggravating hepatitis by prescription of hepatotoxic drugs and because of the availability of alpha-interferon as a potential virus eradicating agent. Also, recognizing fibromyalgia in patients with HCV will prevent misinterpretation of fibromyalgia symptoms as part of the liver disease and will enable the physician to reassure the patient about these symptoms and to alleviate them (Buskila et al., 1997).

**histocompatibility linkage:** A few studies have reported familial aggregation of fibromyalgia (*see* GENETICS), and Yunus (1998) and Yunus et al. (1999) have documented a weak association between fibromyalgia and the human leukocyte antigen (HLA) gene region.

**homeopathy:** Patients with rheumatic syndromes often seek alternative therapies, with homeopathy being one of the most frequent (Jonas et al., 2000). Although homeopathy is one of the most frequently used complementary therapies worldwide, clinical trials involving its effects on fibromyalgia are warranted.

**homocysteine:** Regland et al. (1997) found increased homocysteine levels in the central nervous system in twelve patients fulfilling the criteria for both fibromyalgia and chronic fatigue syndrome. Cerebrospinal homocysteine levels correlated with fatiguability and vitamin B12 levels. Vitamin B12 deficiency causes a deficient remethylation of homocysteine and is, therefore, probably contributing to the increased homocysteine levels found in this patient group.

**hyaluronic acid:** Barkhuizen and Bennett (1999) and Yaron et al. (1997) reported that serum levels of hyaluronic acid, a breakdown product of collagen, in fibromyalgic women were significantly elevated compared to healthy controls and rheumatoid arthritis patients (*see* COLLAGEN).

**hydrocortisone:** Low-dose hydrocortisone injections have been tested for the treatment of chronic fatigue syndrome and fibromyalgia, but more evidence for this therapeutic modality needs to be garnered, and it may only partially benefit a subset of patients (Teitelbaum et al., 1999).

**hyperkalemic periodic paralysis:** Gotze et al. (1998) reported that a forty-three-year-old woman with hyperkalemic periodic paralysis was erroneously diagnosed as having fibromyalgia based on the criteria of the American College of Rheumatology. Her son and three close relatives also had histories of muscle pain and fatigue increasing with age.

**hyperparathyroidism:** The symptoms of hyperparathyroidism are vague and often similar to symptoms of depression, irritable bowel syndrome, fibromyalgia, or stress reaction (Allerheiligen et al., 1998). Hyperparathyroidism is a common cause of hypercalcemia. The hypercalcemia usually is discovered during a routine serum chemistry profile. Often, there has been no previous suspicion of this disorder. In most patients initially believed to be asymptomatic, previously unrecognized symptoms resolve with surgical correction of the disorder.

**hypervigilance:** It has been postulated that the enhanced pain sensitivity in fibromyalgia results from a higher pain magnitude in response to nociceptive stimuli (hyperalgesia) or from a general perceptual amplification of sensations (hypervigilance). A study of twenty fibromyalgia patients by McDermid et al. (1996) supported the hypervigilance model of pain perception in fibromyalgia by documenting that fibromyalgia patients have a heightened sensitivity to pain (e.g., low threshold and tolerance) because of increased attention to external stimulation and a preoccupation with pain sensations. However, no evidence for hypervigilance for innocuous electrocutaneous signals was found in a study of thirty fibromyalgia patients; they did not show superior detection of electrical stimuli either under single or dual task conditions when compared to thirty controls. Also, no differences were found between patients and controls on the body vigilance questionnaire (Peters et al., 2000). Lorenz (1998) also challenged the hypervigilance model by failing to find differences in auditory perception among fibromyalgia patients.

**hypnosis:** Hypnosis is a powerful tool in pain therapy, and fibromyalgia patients experience less pain during hypnotically induced analgesia than during resting wakefulness (Wik et al., 1999). Wik et al. (1999) showed that hypnotic analgesia is associated with a bilaterally increased cerebral blood flow in the orbitofrontal and subcallosial cingulate cortices, the right thalamus, and the left inferior parietal cortex, and bilaterally decreased flow in the cingulate cortex.

**I** **Immunology:** Unlike chronic fatigue syndrome patients, fibromyalgia patients do not show clear evidence of immunological derangements. For instance, in a study of fourteen fibromyalgia patients, Bonaccorso et al. (1998) found no evidence of activation of cell-mediated immunity, and Samborski et al. (1996) found no differences in lymphocyte immunophenotypes (percentage of CD3, CD19, CD4, CD8, CD3/HLA-DR, and CD4/CD45RA) in fibromyalgia patients as compared to healthy controls (*see also* NATURAL KILLER CELLS). Despite the apparent lack of chronic immunological changes in fibromyalgia, several studies have used immunological markers as correlates for fibromyalgia symptomatology or for variables that affect it. In this respect, pain and stiffness in fibromyalgia may be accompanied by a suppression of some aspects of the inflammatory response system (higher sgp130 and lower soluble CD8 serum levels), and the presence of clinically significant depressive symptoms in fibromyalgia is associated with some signs of inflammatory response system activation (higher soluble IL-6 receptor and IL-1 receptor antagonist serum levels) (Maes et al., 1999). Smart et al. (1997) found that fibromyalgia patients who test positive for antinuclear antibodies represent a subgroup of fibromyalgia patients with a more pronounced inflammatory response profile than those patients who test negative for antinuclear antibodies. Samborski et al. (1996) found evidence for allergies in 50 percent of fibromyalgia patients and evidence of CD8 cell suppression of immunoglobulin E production in these patients. Cole et al. (1999) showed that among individuals with functional bowel disease and fibromyalgia, those who were socially inhibited exhibited, under high but not low engagement conditions, significantly increased induration in response to intradermal tetanus toxoid, an observation that indicates heightened delayed-type hypersensitivity response with social inhibition.

**inflammatory bowel disease:** Rheumatological complications of inflammatory bowel disease (Crohn's disease and ulcerative colitis) include peripheral arthritis and spondylitis, and soft tissue rheumatism, specifically fibromyalgia. In a study by Buskila et al. (1999), fibromyalgia was documented in 30 of 113 patients with inflammatory bowel disease (30 percent), specifically in 49 percent of patients with Crohn's disease and 19 percent with ulcerative colitis; in controls, the rate was 0 percent. Subjects with Crohn's disease exhibited more tenderness and reported more frequent and more severe fibromyalgia associated symptoms than subjects with ulcerative colitis. Recognizing fibromyalgia in patients with inflammatory bowel disease will prevent misdiagnosis and ensure correct treatment.

**inflammatory spinal pain:** Patients are said to have inflammatory spinal pain if they fulfill at presentation four of the following five criteria: duration of spinal discomfort for at least three months, spinal morning stiffness, age less than forty, insidious onset of symptoms, and no relief from pain with rest, but improvement with exercise. Inflammatory spinal pain is typical of the spondylarthropathies. Only in a minority of the cases is it found in other rheumatic disorders, such as rheumatoid arthritis, fibromyalgia, infectious spondylitis, or tuberculous spondylitis (Cantini et al., 1998).

**insulin-like growth factor-1:** Some of the clinical features of fibromyalgia resemble the ones described in the adult growth hormone-deficiency syndrome (Leal-Cerro et al., 1999), and serum levels of insulin-like growth factor-1 (IGF-1), also known as somatomedin C, have been found to be decreased in fibromyalgia patients (Bennett et al., 1997), suggesting that disruption of the growth hormone-IGF-1 axis might explain the link between muscle pain and poor sleep. Leal-

Cerro et al. (1999) found that fibromyalgia patients exhibit a marked decrease in spontaneous growth hormone secretion but normal pituitary responsiveness to exogenously administered growth hormone-releasing hormone (GHRH), an observation that suggests the existence of an alteration at the hypothalamic level in the neuroendocrine control of growth hormone and IGF in these patients. Leal-Cerro et al. (1999) also found that growth hormone treatment over four days led to increased IGF-1 and IGF-binding protein-3 (IGFBP3) levels.

Despite the clinical similarities between fibromyalgia and chronic fatigue syndrome (CFS), Bennet et al. (1997) found that serum IGF-1 levels are elevated in the latter syndrome, an observation that suggests that fibromyalgia and CFS may be associated with different abnormalities of sleep and/or of the somatotropic neuroendocrine axis. However, Buchwald et al. (1996) found no differences in serum IGF-1 and IGFBP3 levels among patients with fibromyalgia, CFS, CFS and fibromyalgia, and controls. Jacobsen et al. (1995) and Romano (1996) failed to find major secretory deficiencies of growth hormone and IGF-1 in fibromyalgia. Several factors could contribute to the differences in findings among the studies. For instance, Dessein et al. (1999) reported that IGF-1 serum levels were lower in obese patients as compared to nonobese patients.

In terms of the origin of the relationship between low IGF-1 levels and pain and sleep problems in fibromyalgia, Older et al. (1998) found that three nights of delta-wave sleep interruption caused no significant lowering of pain thresholds or serum IGF-1 in healthy volunteers, which caused them to conclude that the low levels of IGF-1 seen in fibromyalgia patients may result from chronic rather than acute delta-wave sleep interruption or may be dependent on factors other than disturbances of delta-wave sleep. In support of the latter possibility, Jacobsen et al. (1995) reported that although fibromyalgia patients had more sleep problems than controls, no major differences in IGF-1 levels were apparent.

**interferon-alpha:** In two reports, Russell, Michalek, et al. (1999) and Russell, Vipraio, et al. (1999) documented that daily sublingual interferon-alpha at different doses (15, 50, or 150 IU) was not associated with significant improvement or adverse events in fibromyalgia patients. Interferon-alpha is used for the treatment of viral hepatitis C-associated disease.

**interstitial cystitis:** Interstitial cystitis is a relatively uncommon disorder characterized by pain in the bladder and pelvic region, typically accompanied by urinary urgency and frequency (Clauw et al., 1997). Although genitourinary and musculoskeletal symptoms predominate in interstitial cystitis and fibromyalgia, respectively, both disorders share a number of features, including similar symptomatology (diffusely increased peripheral nociception and increased pain sensitivity), demographics, natural history, aggravating factors, overlapping conditions (allergies, irritable bowel syndrome), and efficacious therapy (Clauw et al., 1997). In comparison to the general population, individuals with interstitial cystitis are 100 times more likely to have inflammatory bowel disease and 30 times more likely to have systemic lupus erythematosus (Alagiri et al., 1997).

**intramuscular stimulation:** In retrospective analyses of two and six patients, Chu (2000a,b) showed that automated twitch-obtaining intramuscular stimulation (ATOIMS) and electrical twitch-obtaining intramuscular stimulation (ETOIMS) methods are promising in the control of radiculopathy-related myofascial pain and fibromyalgia. Reduction of mechanical tension through muscle relaxation is the proposed basis for the pain relief.

**irritable bowel syndrome:** Irritable bowel syndrome and fibromyalgia are considered chronic syndromes of altered visceral and somatic perception, respectively (Chang, 1998; Chang et al., 2000; Chun et al., 1999; Mayer et al., 1998; Sivri et al., 1996). As many as 70 percent of patients with fibromyalgia complain of the symptoms of irritable bowel syndrome, and approximately 35 percent of patients with irritable bowel syndrome also have fibromyalgia (Barton et al., 1999; Chang, 1998). The diagnostic criteria of fibromyalgia syndrome include irritable bowel syndrome, and, hence, a common etiopathophysiology has been suggested (Azpiroz et al., 2000; Sperber, Atzmon, et al., 1999; Sperber, Carmel, et al., 1999). Similar to fibromyalgia, a large proportion of irritable bowel syndrome patients also complain of other functional disorders, such as headache, noncardiac chest pain, low back pain, sicca complex, and dysuria (Chang, 1998; Mayer et al., 1998). Sperber, Atzmon, et al. (1999), Sperber, Carmel, et al., (1999), Sperber et al. (2000), and Chang et al. (2000) found that patients with both irritable bowel syndrome and fibromyalgia have increased severity of symptoms. However, both hypervigilance and somatic hypoalgesia contribute to the altered somatic perception in irritable bowel syndrome patients, while comorbidity with fibromyalgia results in somatic hyperalgesia in irritable bowel syndrome patients (Chang, 1998; Chang et al., 2000). Another distinctive feature was pointed out by the study of Chun et al. (1999), which found that although patients with fibromyalgia and sphincter of Oddi dysfunction, type III, share many demographic and psychosocial characteristics with patients with irritable bowel syndrome (Chun et al., 1999), the latter have significantly lower rectal pain thresholds and increased levels of psychologic distress compared to controls.

**J** **joint hypermobility:** The estimated prevalence of generalized hypermobility in the adult population is 5 to 15 percent, and hypermobile individuals may be predisposed to soft tissue trauma and subsequent musculoskeletal pain and rheumatism (Hudson et al., 1995, 1998). Some patients who have clinical symptoms of fibromyalgia but do not exactly meet the American College of Rheumatology criteria could in fact have joint hypermobility, and these patients may be misdiagnosed as having fibromyalgia. Widespread pain is associated with joint hypermobility in women under age fifty, and fibromyalgia and joint hypermobility may coexist (Acasuso-Diaz and Collantes-Estevez, 1998; Fitzcharles, 2000; Klemp, 1997). Karaaslan et al. (2000) reported that the frequency of joint hypermobility was 8 percent in patients with fibromyalgia and 6 percent in subjects without fibromyalgia. Acasuso-Diaz et al. (1998) and Hudson et al. (1995) reported that 27 to 30 percent of fibromyalgia patients suffered joint hyperlaxity. In a review of the medical charts of 2,500 female patients seen in a rheumatology practice, Lai et al. (2000) documented that joint hypermobility was independently associated with both fibromyalgia and with breast implantation, but fibromyalgia and breast implantation were not found to be independently associated with each other.

**juvenile fibromyalgia:** The frequency of chronic pain syndromes in pediatric rheumatology has increased over the past twenty-five years. Diagnosis is complex: underlying organic illness, somatization, and growing pains are all possibilities (Cassidy, 1998). Fibromyalgia has also been recognized in children and adolescents as juvenile fibromyalgia (JF) (Buskila, 1996; Clark et al., 1998; Kulig, 1991; Sherry, 1997; Tayag-Kier et al., 2000). Juvenile rheumatoid arthritis (JRA) and juvenile fibromyalgia can coexist (Schikler, 2000). For the patient with an initial diagnosis of either JRA or JF whose clinical response to therapy is not in keeping with expectations or physical examination findings or whose clinical course worsens without explanation, reevaluation to determine if JF in the JRA patient has developed or JRA in the JF patient has emerged is warranted.

The clinical spectrum of fibromyalgia in children (diffuse aching, headaches, sleep disturbances, and, less commonly, stiffness, subjective joint swelling, fatigue, abdominal pain, joint hypermobility, dizziness, and depression) is similar to that of adults but with better outcomes (Gedalia et al., 2000; Mikkelsson, Salminen, et al., 1997; Mikkelsson, Sourander, et al., 1997; Mikkelsson, 1999; Rusy et al., 1999; Sieb et al., 1997; Siegel et al., 1998). Tayag-Kier et al. (2000) also demonstrated, in sixteen children and adolescents with JF, abnormalities in sleep architecture, including periodic limb movement in sleep, similar to those seen in adult fibromyalgia patients. However, Breau et al. (1999) consider that fibromyalgia and chronic fatigue syndrome may be related in children and may not be duplicates of the adult disorders; that psychological and psychosocial factors are unlikely contributors to the etiology of these disorders; and that the evidence is increasingly pointing to a role for genetic factors in their etiology. Roizenblatt et al. (1997) reported a significant concordance of fibromyalgia diagnosis and significant correlations between polysomnographic indexes, sleep anomalies, and pain manifestations in children and their mothers.

Gedalia et al. (2000) reported that active exercise programs seem to correlate with better outcomes in JF. Kujala et al. (1999) point out that, in addition to its likely long-term health benefits, vigorous physical activity causes musculoskeletal pains during adolescence, which should be considered as a confounder in epidemiological studies on fibromyalgia and related issues. In terms of other factors that affect JF symptomatology, Schanberg et al. (1998) found that family environment and parental pain history may be related to how children cope with JF. Behavioral interventions targeting the family may improve the long-term functional status of children with JF (Haavet and

Grunfeld, 1997; Schanberg et al., 1996). In this respect, Reid et al. (1997) point out that disability among children with fibromyalgia or JRA is a function of the children's psychological adjustment and physical state, and of the parents' physical state and method of coping with pain.

 **keratoconjunctivitis sicca:** Patients with fibromyalgia often describe the presence of dry eyes and other ocular symptoms (Barton et al., 1999), and it has been claimed that a subgroup of fibromyalgia patients might have features suggestive of primary Sjogren's syndrome (*see also* SJOGREN'S SYNDROME). However, Gunaydin et al. (1999) found that chronic blepharitis and the use of tricyclic antidepressants may play a role in developing keratoconjunctivitis sicca among fibromyalgia patients, and the rate of the latter disorder does not increase in fibromyalgia patients who probably have objective ocular findings comparable with the normal population.

**ketamine:** Graven-Nielsen et al. (2000) showed that mechanisms involved in referred pain, temporal summation, muscular hyperalgesia, and muscle pain at rest were attenuated by intravenous injection of the N-methyl-D-aspartate (NMDA) receptor antagonist ketamine (0.3 mg/kg, Ketalar) in fibromyalgia patients. Whether the latter effect is specific for fibromyalgia patients or a general phenomena in painful musculoskeletal disorders is not known. A single sub-anaesthetic dose of ketamine causes a long-term depression of pain intensity in some, but not in all, patients suffering chronic pain (Oye et al., 1996). This effect is distinctly different from the short-lasting (10 to 30 minutes) analgesic effect in cases of acute nociceptive pain. The long-term depression of the intensity of chronic pain states may be due to a reversal of NMDA receptor-dependent long-term potentiation of synapses in central pain pathways.

***Klebsiella:*** No evidence for the existence of disease-specific *Klebsiella* species was obtained by Toivanen et al. (1999) when analyzing, either separately or simultaneously according to somatic serotypes (O groups), capsular (K) serotypes, and biochemically identified species, feces from 187 ankylosing spondylitis patients and 195 fibromyalgia or rheumatoid arthritis patients.

 **laser therapy:** Longo et al. (1997) showed that two-thirds of 846 patients with fibromyositic rheumatisms, untreatable with other therapies, responded to therapy with defocalized laser beams (analgesic and antiphlogistic effects). This form of therapy needs standardization.

**leiomyosarcoma:** A retroperitoneal leiomyosarcoma was reported in a patient who had been diagnosed with fibromyalgia (De Tomas Palacios et al., 1995).

**lidocaine:** The antinociceptive effects of systemically administered local anesthetics have been shown in various conditions, such as neuralgia, polyneuropathy, fibromyalgia, and postoperative pain (Koppert et al., 1998). Injection of low-dose local anesthetics, such as lidocaine, are also useful in pain states, such as fibromyalgia, which are dominated by hyperalgesia. In this respect, increasing painfulness during sustained pinching has been attributed to excitation and simultaneous sensitization of particular Adelta- and C-nociceptors. This hyperalgesic mechanism seems to be particularly sensitive to low concentrations of injected lidocaine (Koppert et al., 1998). In contrast to the latter observation, Scudds et al. (1995) found no efficacy in pain reduction when using 4 percent topical lidocaine in sphenopalatine blocks in forty-two fibromyalgia patients and nineteen with myofascial pain syndrome. Moreover, Figuerola et al. (1998) showed an increase in plasma metenkephalin levels ten minutes after either local injection of lidocaine hydrochloride, local injection of saline, or dry needling.

**light treatment:** In a randomized ten-week crossover study comparing the effects of four weeks of "visible electromagnetic fields" (light condition; mean 4,750 lux, SD 2,337 lux) to four weeks of "nonvisible electromagnetic fields" (no light condition) in fourteen fibromyalgia patients reporting seasonality of symptoms, Pearl et al. (1996) found no significant differences between the light and no-light conditions on pain, mood, or sleep. However, Tabeeva et al.

(1998) reported that phototherapy of fibromyalgia patients was associated with an increase of total sleep duration, and a decrease of the time of falling asleep, the latent period of the phase of fast sleep, activated movement index, intensivity of movements, and arousal time during sleep. A distinction should be made between fibromyalgia and seasonal affective disorder.

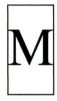 **magnesium:** In a study of ninety-seven patients, Moorkens et al. (1997) found no association between magnesium deficiency and chronic fatigue syndrome or fibromyalgia. However, serum magnesium levels were significantly lower in those patients with spasmophilia. Eisinger et al. (1996) also failed to find magnesium deficiency in twenty-five fibromyalgia patients studied.

**massage:** A study by Brattberg (1999) of forty-eight individuals diagnosed with fibromyalgia (twenty-three in the treatment group and twenty-five in the reference group) showed that a series of fifteen treatments with connective tissue massage conveys a pain-relieving effect of 37 percent, reduces depression and the use of analgesics, and positively affects quality of life. The treatment effects appeared gradually during the ten-week treatment period. Three months after the treatment period, about 30 percent of the pain-relieving effect was gone, and six months after the treatment period, pain was back to about 90 percent of the baseline value.

**masticatory myofascial pain:** Cimino et al. (1998) reported several similarities between fibromyalgia and masticatory myofascial pain in forty-six patients affected by craniomandibular disorders, the most striking of which were pain during mandibular function, articular noises, and headache. Both groups had similar mean scores of muscle pain upon palpation, mean values of active mouth opening, and mean values of passive opening. Cimino and colleagues recommend that the physician should be alert to the need to conduct interdisciplinary evaluations in the diagnosis and management of fibromyalgia and of masticatory myofascial pain.

**medicinal baths:** In a randomized, comparative, and investigator-blinded study of thirty outpatients with generalized fibromyalgia undergoing therapy consisting of either ten whirl baths with plain water or with the addition of pine oil or valerian, Ammer and Melnizky (1999) found that plain-water baths modify the pain intensity while medicinal baths improve well-being and sleep.

**melatonin:** Desynchronization of circadian systems has been postulated in the etiology of fibromyalgia. The pineal hormone melatonin is involved in synchronizing circadian systems, and the use of exogenous melatonin has become widespread in patients with fibromyalgia and chronic fatigue syndrome (Webb, 1998). However, Korszun et al. (1999) found that although nighttime plasma melatonin levels were significantly higher in fibromyalgia patients compared to controls, there were no differences in the timing of cortisol and melatonin secretory patterns and no internal desynchronization of the two rhythms in fibromyalgia patients compared to controls. Raised plasma melatonin concentrations have been documented in several other conditions that are associated with dysregulation of neuroendocrine axes, and increased melatonin levels may represent a marker of increased susceptibility to stress-induced hypothalamic disruptions (*see also* NEUROENDOCRINOLOGY). Although the latter data indicate that there is no rationale for melatonin replacement therapy in fibromyalgia patients, in a preliminary four-week pilot study of treatment with melatonin (3 mg at bedtime) in nineteen fibromyalgia patients, Citera et al. (2000) reported significant improvements after thirty days in median values for the tender point count and severity of pain at selected points, patient and physician global assessments, and sleep. Also, unlike Korszun et al. (1999), Wikner et al. (1998), found a 31 percent lower nighttime melatonin secretion in eight fibromyalgia patients as compared to healthy subjects and proposed that this deficiency may contribute to impaired sleep at night, fatigue during the day, and changed pain perception. However, Press et al. (1998) found that nocturnal urine 6-sulphatoxymelatonin levels were similar in thirty-nine fibromyalgia patients and controls.

**mitochondrial myopathy:** Mitochondrial myopathy can also mimic fibromyalgia and should be included in the differential (Benito-Leon et al., 1996; Villanova et al., 1999).

**moclobemide:** A four-center, twelve-week study by Hannonen et al. (1998) of 130 female fibromyalgia patients without psychiatric disorders showed that although moclobemide (450 to 600 mg) improved pain, the improvement was invalidated by the poor success of the drug with regard to sleep.

**motor cortical dysfunction:** In a study of thirteen fibromyalgia patients using single and double magnetic stimulation, Salerno et al. (2000) demonstrated motor cortical dysfunction involving excitatory and inhibitory mechanisms, an observation that supports the hypothesis of aberrant central pain mechanisms. Similar observations were made in five rheumatoid arthritis patients, a finding which suggests that the lesions were not specific and could be related to chronic pain disorders within the central nervous system. Ivanichev and Starosel'tseva (2000) proposed a model based on proprioceptive desafferentation which promotes disinhibition of neurons and formation of the generators of pathologically increased irritation with positive feedback on rubro-segmental, pallido-thalamic, strio-piramidal, and parietal-premotor levels of the construction of the movement. Moreover, based on a comparison of the movement disorders in fibromyalgia patients to those found in akinetic syndromes that are secondary to disturbances in the functions of the cortico-thalamo-nigro-striatal system and associated areas, Burgunder (1998) proposes that since basal ganglia also play a role in pain, a comparative study of their involvement in movement disorders and nociception seems to be fruitful, especially in devising new therapeutic strategies.

**mud packs:** Bellometti and Galzigna (1999) reported that mud packs together with antidepressant treatment (trazodone) are able to influence the hypothalamic-pituitary axis, stimulating increased levels of adrenocorticotropic hormone, cortisol, and beta-endorphin serum levels. The discharge of corticoids in the blood and the increase in beta-endorphin serum levels are followed by a reduction in pain symptoms, which is closely related to an improvement in ability, depression, and quality of life. It seems that the synergistic association between a pharmacological treatment (trazodone) and mud packs acts by helping the physiological responses to achieve homeostasis and to rebalance the stress response system.

**muscle abnormalities:** An assessment of maximal and explosive strength characteristics of the leg muscles and a comparison of acute neuromuscular fatigue during heavy resistance loading and short-term recovery from fatigue failed to demonstrate lower dynamic or isometric muscle strength characteristics in eleven premenopausal women with fibromyalgia as compared to twelve matched healthy female controls (Hakkinen et al., 2000). The latter observations strongly support normal muscle structure and neuromuscular function in fibromyalgia patients (Simms, 1996).

Some earlier studies disagree with the latter conclusion of normal structure and muscle function in fibromyalgia. For instance, Pongratz and Spath (1998) found that the most common morphological finding in muscle biopsies in long-standing fibromyalgia is type II fiber atrophy, a change that can be found in many other conditions, such as disuse atrophy, affections of the corticospinal tracts, steroid atrophy, and other different neuromuscular disorders. Pongratz and Spath (1998) also found that an increase in lipid droplets and a slight proliferation of mitochondria in type I muscle fibers correlated with the duration of fibromyalgia and that some fibromyalgia patients with ragged red fibers, which histochemically show a pronounced accumulation of lipids and mitochondria and single fiber defects of cytochrome-c-oxidase, had deletions of the mitochondrial genome. However, although Norregaard (1998), Norregaard et al. (1995), and Borman et al. (1999) reported reduced quadriceps muscle strength and submaximal aerobic performance in fibromyalgia patients, there was no relation between the decreased muscle performance and clinical findings, including pain severity, number of tender points, and duration of the symptoms. Graven-Nielsen et al. (1997) suggest that modulation of muscle activity by muscle pain could be controlled via inhibition of muscles agonistic to the movement and/or excitation of muscles antagonistic to the movement.

Simms (1996) points out that the studies which indicated morphologic abnormalities in fibromyalgia patients had major problems with patient selection and lacked adequate control groups. Jacobsen (1998) and Olsen and Park (1998) reinforced that there are no signs of specific muscle pathology in fibromyalgia and that alterations in muscle function may reflect effects of deconditioning or inhibition of contraction due to spinal or supraspinal mechanisms. Moreover, phosphorus magnetic resonance spectroscopy has been used in the investigation of muscle energy metabolism (Argov et al., 2000; Strobel et al., 1997) and, although Sprott et al. (2000) found increases in the levels of phosphodiesterase and inorganic phosphate in the fibromyalgic muscle tissue of fifteen patients as compared to seventeen healthy controls, the latter authors suggest that the latter metabolic differences may have been related to weakness and fatigue in the fibromyalgia patients, and they do not fully explain the fibromyalgia symptoms. Park et al. (1998) also studied the biochemical status of muscle in eleven fibromyalgia patients and showed that patients had significantly lower than normal phosphocreatinine and ATP levels and phosphocreatinine to inorganic phosphate ratios in the quadriceps muscles during rest, metabolic abnormalities that are consistent with weakness and fatigue. Studies of muscle blood flow and motor unit recruitment also demonstrate abnormalities that can be explained by deconditioning alone (Simms, 1996; Vestergaard-Poulsen et al., 1995). Thorsteinsdottir et al. (1998) found no difference in ubiquinone concentration of muscles and blood in fibromyalgia patients and healthy controls.

Based on the observation of an increased sensitivity of the flare reaction in fibromyalgia patients, Sann and Pierau (1998) suggest that the hyperalgesia characteristic of fibromyalgia might be partly due to altered functions of C-fiber nociceptors. Local efferent functions of C-fiber nociceptors, such as vasodilation and the axon reflex flare reaction, are mediated via a local release of substance P, neurokinin A, and calcitonin gene-related peptide (CGRP) from the peripheral ending. CGRP is the main mediator of the capsaicin-induced flare reaction in mammalian skin. The latter theory of the genesis of pain in fibromyalgia syndrome is that excessive muscle tension leads to increased excitability of nociceptors in muscle, which in turn leads to muscle hypertension and chronic pain. Furthermore, defective sympathetic control (Wachter et al., 1996) is proposed to result in disturbed microcirculation and nociceptor excitation. In aggregate, however, studies using EMG techniques show no evidence of excessive muscle tension or defective sympathetic nervous function (Simms, 1996). Therefore, although muscular pain has been a central feature of fibromyalgia syndrome (Henriksson et al., 1996), controlled studies of muscle fail to support a convincing role for muscle in the pathophysiology of the condition. Muscle tenderness in fibromyalgia cannot be explained on the basis of primary muscle abnormalities, either structural or functional.

**mycoplasma:** More than 60 percent of patients with chronic fatigue syndrome/fibromyalgia syndrome, as compared to 15 percent in controls, have mycoplasmal blood infections, such as *Mycoplasma fermentans* infection (Choppa et al., 1998; Nasralla et al., 1999). The role of *Mycoplasma* as an etiological agent for fibromyalgia or chronic fatigue syndrome remains controversial.

**myoadenylate deaminase deficiency:** Marin and Connick (1997) described a patient who was treated unsuccessfully for fibromyalgia for many years and who ultimately was diagnosed with a rare benign skeletal muscle metabolic disorder caused by myoadenylate deaminase deficiency.

**myofascial pain syndrome:** Myofascial pain syndrome (MPS) is a very common localized—sometimes also polytopic—painful musculoskeletal condition associated with trigger points for which, however, diagnostic criteria established in well-designed studies are still lacking (Cimino et al., 1998; Pongratz and Spath, 1998). Fibromyalgia should be included in the differential diagnosis for myofascial pain of the masticatory or facial muscles (Aronoff, 1998; Bernstein, 1997; Bohr, 1996; Dao et al., 1997; Fishbain and Rosomoff, 1996; Galer, 1997; Gantz and Fukuda, 1997; Goldenberg, 1996; Long, 1997; Nye, 1997; Perle, 1996; Romano, 1997).

Harden et al. (2000) surveyed American Pain Society members, and 88.5 percent of respondents reported that MPS is a legitimate diagnosis, with 81 percent describing MPS as distinct from fibromyalgia. The only signs and symptoms described as essential to the diagnosis of MPS by greater than 50 percent of the sample were regional location, presence of trigger points, and a normal neurologic examination. Regarding the signs and symptoms considered to be essential or associated with MPS, more than 80 percent of respondents agreed on regional location, trigger points, normal neurologic examination, reduced pain with local anesthetic or "spray and stretch," taut bands, tender points, palpable nodules, muscle ropiness, decreased range of motion, pain exacerbated by stress, and regional pain described as "dull," "achy," or "deep." Sensory or reflex abnormalities, scar tissue, and most test results were considered to be irrelevant to the diagnosis of MPS by a large proportion of the respondents.

Some patients may exhibit both MPS and fibromyalgia (Dao et al., 1998). For instance, of the 162 female participants with a history of myofascial face pain, Raphael et al. (2000) found that thirty-eight (23.5 percent) reported a history of fibromyalgia. Patients who have myofascial face pain and a history of widespread pain suggestive of fibromyalgia are likely to have more persistent and debilitating myofascial face pain and to have higher rates of depression and somatization symptoms than those who have no history of widespread pain. Raphael and Marbach (2000) also found reduced fertility among women with myofascial face pain, but this was restricted to those who self-report a history of fibromyalgia.

The most important criteria for differential diagnosis are the presence of tender points (TePs) and widespread, nonspecific, soft tissue pain in fibromyalgia, compared with regional and characteristic referred pain patterns with discrete muscular trigger points (TrPs) and taut bands of skeletal muscle in MPS. Myofascial TrPs are found within a taut band of skeletal muscle and have a characteristic "nodular" texture upon palpation. TrPs are thought to develop after trauma, overuse, or prolonged spasm of muscles. Local treatment applied to TePs is ineffective, yet specific treatment of TrPs is often dramatically effective.

Fibromyalgia is a systemic disease process, apparently caused by dysfunction of the limbic system and/or neuroendocrine axis, and often requiring a multidisciplinary treatment approach, while MPS is a condition that arises from the referred pain and muscle dysfunction caused by TrPs, which often respond to manual treatment methods such as ischemic compression and various specific stretching techniques (Schneider, 1995).

 **natural killer cells:** Natural killer (NK) cells are mostly large granular lymphocytes and are constitutively cytocidal against tumor-transformed and virus-infected cells, an activity that does not require immunization (Patarca et al., 1995). Although several studies revealed impaired NK cell function in chronic fatigue syndrome patients as assessed by cytotoxic activity against K562 target cells (Barker et al., 1994; DuBois, 1986; Gupta and Vayuvegula, 1991; Kibler et al.,

1985; Klimas et al., 1990; Morrison et al., 1991; Ojo-Amaise et al., 1994; See et al., 1997; Straus et al., 1985; Whiteside and Friberg, 1998), Russell et al. (1999) found no difference in the natural killer cell activity or response to interferon-alpha in fibromyalgia patients as compared to controls.

NK cell activity is known to be decreased by stress and, partly replicating previous data in healthy volunteers, Lekander et al. (2000) found that natural killer cell activity in fibromyalgia patients correlated negatively with right hemisphere activity in the secondary somatosensory and motor cortices as well as the thalamus. Moreover, natural killer cell activity was negatively and bilaterally related to activity in the posterior cingulate cortex. The latter findings illustrate that immune parameters are related to activity in brain areas involved in pain perception, emotion, and attention (Lekander et al., 2000).

**neck support:** Ambrogio et al. (1998) found inconclusive evidence in a study of thirty-five fibromyalgia patients who tried three types of neck support (Shape of Sleep pillow, two neck ruffs with one standard pillow, and a single standard pillow). However, from a patient's perspective, neck support is an important part of a comprehensive physiotherapy program.

**nerve growth factor:** Giovengo et al. (1999) found elevated levels of the neuropeptide nerve growth factor in the cerebrospinal fluid of primary, but not secondary, fibromyalgia patients (41.8 +/–12.7 pg/mL versus 9.1 +/–4.1 pg/mL in controls), an observation that reinforces the notion of a central mechanism in the pathogenesis of fibromyalgia.

**neuroendocrinology:** The neuroendocrine axes are essential physiologic systems that allow for communication between the brain and the body (Crofford, 1998a,b; Morand et al., 1996). Interconnections among the neuroendocrine axes coordinate regulation of these systems in both a positive and negative fashion (Crofford, 1998a,b). Changes in neuroendocrine transmitters such as serotonin, substance P, growth hormone, and cortisol suggest that dysregulation of the autonomic and neuroendocrine systems are associated with fibromyalgia (Bellometti and Galzigna, 1999; Bradley et al., 2000; Clauw and Chrousos, 1997; Crofford et al., 1996; Dessein et al., 2000; Griep et al.,

1998; Heim et al., 2000; Millea and Holloway, 2000; Pillemer et al., 1997; Russell, 1998; Scott and Dinan, 1999). Almost all of the hormonal feedback mechanisms controlled by the hypothalamus are altered in fibromyalgia, as evinced by elevated basal values of adrenocorticotropic hormone (ACTH), follicle-stimulating hormone (FSH), and cortisol, as well as lowered basal values of insulin-like growth factor-1 (IGF-1, somatomedin C), free triiodothyronine (FT3), and estrogen (Bennett et al., 1997; Clauw and Chrousos, 1997; Griep et al., 1998; Neeck, 2000; Riedel et al., 1998). In fibromyalgia patients, the systemic administration of corticotropin-releasing hormone (CRH), growth hormone-releasing hormone (GHRH), thyrotropin-releasing hormone (TRH), and luteinizing hormone-releasing hormone (LHRH) leads to increased secretion of ACTH and prolactin, whereas the degree to which thyroid-stimulating hormone (TSH) can be stimulated is reduced (Neeck and Riedel, 1999; Netter and Hennig, 1998; Riedel et al., 1998). The stimulation of the hypophysis with LHRH in female fibromyalgia patients during their follicular phase results in a significantly reduced luteinizing hormone response (Neeck and Riedel, 1999; Riedel et al., 1998). Based on the latter observations, it has been proposed that the alterations in set points of hormonal regulation that are typical for fibromyalgia patients can be explained as a primary stress activation of hypothalamic CRH neurons caused by chronic pain or other factors (Crofford and Demitrack, 1996; Lentjes et al., 1997; Neeck, 2000; Netter and Hennig, 1998; Oye et al., 1996; Stanton, 1999; Torpy and Chrousos, 1996; Winfield, 1999). In addition to the stimulation of pituitary ACTH secretion, CRH activates somatostatin on the hypothalamic level, which in turn inhibits the release of GH and TSH at the hypophyseal level. The lowered estrogen levels could be accounted for both via an inhibitory effect of the CRH on the hypothalamic release of LHRH or via a direct CRH-mediated inhibition of the FSH-stimulated estrogen production in the ovary. Serotonin (5HT), precursors such as tryptophan (5HTP), drugs that release 5HT or act directly on 5HT receptors stimulate the hypothalamic-pituitary-adrenal (HPA) axis, indicating a stimulatory serotonergic influence on HPA axis function. Therefore, activation of the HPA axis may reflect an elevated serotonergic tonus in the central nervous system of fibromyalgia patients. Defects in the HPA axis have also been observed in autoimmune and rheumatic diseases, chronic inflammatory disease, and chronic fatigue syndrome

(Anisman et al., 1996; Crofford et al., 1996; Crofford and Demitrack, 1996; Demitrack, 1997; Demitrack and Crofford, 1998; Scott and Dinan, 1999; Torpy and Chrousos, 1996).

Administration of interleukin (IL)-6 (3 µg/kg of body weight subcutaneously), a cytokine capable of stimulating CRH, to thirteen female fibromyalgia patients yielded exaggerated norepinephrine (NE) responses and heart rate increases, as well as delayed ACTH release (Torpy et al., 2000). The latter observations are consistent with a defect in hypothalamic CRH neuronal function and abnormal regulation of the sympathetic nervous system. The excessive heart rate response after IL-6 injection in fibromyalgia patients may be unrelated to the increase in NE, or it may reflect an alteration in the sensitivity of cardiac beta-adrenoceptors to NE. These responses to a physiologic stressor support the notion that fibromyalgia may represent a primary disorder of the stress system (Torpy et al., 2000).

Not all studies agree with the assessment of endocrine function described previously. For instance, in a study of fifteen premenopausal women with fibromyalgia, Samborski et al. (1996) failed to find significant differences in the levels of ACTH, substance P, and TSH in fibromyalgia patients compared to controls. Adler et al. (1999) reported that although twenty-four-hour urinary free cortisol levels and diurnal patterns of ACTH and cortisol were normal, as also found by Maes et al. (1998), there was a significant (approximately 30 percent) reduction in the ACTH and epinephrine responses to hypoglycemia in women with fibromyalgia compared with controls. Prolactin, norepinephrine, cortisol, and dehydroepiandrosterone responses to hypoglycemia were similar in the two study groups. In subjects with fibromyalgia, the epinephrine response to hypoglycemia correlated inversely with overall health status as measured by the fibromyalgia impact questionnaire. Adler et al. (1999) concluded that fibromyalgia patients have an impaired ability to activate the hypothalamic-pituitary portion of the hypothalamic-pituitary-adrenal (HPA) axis as well as the sympathoadrenal system, leading to reduced ACTH and epinephrine responses to hypoglycemia.

Hapidou and Rollman (1998) reported that the number of tender points identified by palpation was greater in the follicular (postmenstrual) phase of the cycle as compared to the luteal (intermenstrual) phase in normally cycling women but not in users of oral contraceptives. Although the latter and other studies mentioned suggest that sex hormones have a role in fibromyalgia symptomatology

(Akkus et al., 2000; Anderberg, 2000), and Raphael and Marbach (2000) found reduced fecundity among women with myofascial face pain who also reported a history of fibromyalgia, a study by Korszun et al. (2000) of nine premenopausal women with fibromyalgia or eight with chronic fatigue syndrome found no indication of abnormal gonadotropin secretion or gonadal steroid levels (no significant differences in follicle-stimulating hormones, progesterone, or estradiol levels in patients versus controls, and no significant differences in pulsatile secretion of luteinizing hormone).

There is little direct information as to how the specific HPA axis perturbations seen in fibromyalgia can be related to the major symptomatic manifestations of pain, fatigue, sleep disturbance, and psychological distress. Interventions providing symptomatic improvement in patients with fibromyalgia and CFS can directly or indirectly affect the HPA axis. These interventions include exercise, tricyclic antidepressants, and selective serotonin reuptake inhibitors (Crofford, 1998a,b). Moreover, in a study of thirty-six fibromyalgic women patients (with forty pregnancies total), Ostensen et al. (1997) found that all women described worsening fibromyalgia symptoms during pregnancy, with the last trimester experienced as the worst period. A new change of fibromyalgia symptoms within six months after delivery was reported for thirty-seven of the forty pregnancies, to the better in four and to the worse in thirty-three cases, resulting in a prolonged sick leave for fourteen patients. An increase in depression and anxiety was a prominent problem in the postpartum period. Fibromyalgia had no adverse effect on the outcome of pregnancy or the health of the neonate. In the majority of fibromyalgia patients, hormonal changes connected with abortion, use of hormonal contraceptives, and breast-feeding did not modulate symptom severity. A premenstrual worsening of symptoms was recorded by 72 percent of the patients. Comparing the twenty-six patients who had borne children during disease with eighteen patients who had all their children before the onset of fibromyalgia revealed a negative effect of pregnancy and the postpartum period of fibromyalgia and increased functional impairment and disability in the twenty-six patients (Ostensen et al., 1997).

**neurogenic inflammation:** Enestrom et al. (1997) found that skin biopsies from twenty-five fibromyalgia patients had significantly higher values of immunoglobulin (Ig)G deposits in the dermis and vessel walls, showed a higher reactivity for collagen III, and had a higher mean number of mast cells. There was a correlation between the percentage of damaged/degranulated mast cells and the individual IgG immunofluorescence scores. These findings support the hypothesis of neurogenic inflammation involvement in fibromyalgia (*see also* CHEMICAL INTOLERANCE).

**neuroimaging:** Mountz et al. (1995) reported that regional cerebral blood flow (rCBF) in the left and right hemithalami or the left and right heads of the caudate nucleus is significantly lower in women with fibromyalgia than in normal controls. Compared with controls, the women with fibromyalgia also were characterized by significantly lower cortical rCBF and lower pain threshold levels at both tender points and control points. San Pedro et al. (1998) confirmed the findings of lower rCBF and its relationship to pain in fibromyalgia patients. The latter findings support the hypothesis that abnormal pain perception in women with fibromyalgia may result from a functional abnormality within the central nervous system (Yang et al., 1999).

**neuropeptide Y:** Crofford et al. (1996) initially found that the plasma levels of neuropeptide Y (NPY), a peptide colocalized with norepinephrine in the sympathetic nervous system, are low in fibromyalgia patients (Crofford et al., 1996), while in a more recent report Anderberg et al. (1999) found that NPY levels were significantly elevated in fibromyalgia patients compared to the controls. Several factors affect NPY levels. For instance, Anderberg et al. (1999) reported that NPY levels are higher during the luteal phase, and NPY levels correlate with anxiety but not depression. Fibromyalgia patients may, therefore, have an altered activity in the NPY system, most likely due to prolonged and/or repeated stress, and may also be affected by the hormonal state and time of the menstrual cycle.

**nociceptin:** Anderberg et al. (1998) showed that the levels of the neuropeptide nociceptin were lower in fibromyalgia patients than in controls, a finding that may be linked to other neuroendocrine abnormalities reported for fibromyalgia patients (*see* NEUROENDOCRINOLOGY).

**nonsteroidal anti-inflammatory drugs (NSAIDs):** Through a mailed questionnaire survey of 1,799 patients with osteoarthritis, rheumatoid arthritis, or fibromyalgia who were participating in a long-term outcome study, Wolfe et al. (2000) found a considerable and statistically significant preference for NSAIDs compared with acetaminophen among different groups of rheumatic disease patients. Although this preference decreased slightly with age and was less pronounced in osteoarthritis patients, the preference was noted among all categories of patients and was not altered by disease severity. Wolfe et al. (2000) concluded that if safety and cost are not issues there would hardly ever be a reason to recommend acetaminophen over NSAIDs, since patients generally preferred NSAIDs and fewer than 14 percent preferred acetaminophen. Vachtenheim (1995) also reported on the efficacy of a nonsteroidal anti-inflammatory ointment, Mobilisin, which contains flufenamic acid, in fibromyalgia patients. If safety and costs are issues, then the recommendation of the American College of Rheumatology that acetaminophen be tried first seems correct, since 38.2 percent found acetaminophen to be as effective or more effective than NSAIDs (Wolfe et al., 2000).

**nursing:** Nurses can enhance patients' quality of life by helping them to cope with pain, establish sleep patterns, take exercise, manage stress, improve concentration and memory, and fight isolation (Edmands et al., 1999; Ryan, 1995).

O

**omega-3 fatty acids:** As for other rheumatic diseases, Ozgocmen et al. (2000) reported that omega-3 fatty acids may also be useful in the treatment of fibromyalgia.

**opioids:** Opioids are prescribed for the management of pain associated with fibromyalagia. Quang-Cantagrel et al. (2000) showed that if a patient receiving chronic opioid therapy experiences an intolerable side effect or if the drug is ineffective, changing to a different opioid may result in a lessening or elimination of the side effect and/or improved analgesia. In terms of which opioid to prescribe, Quijada-Carrera et al. (1996) reported that treatment with tenoxicam (20 mg) plus bromazepan (3 mg) can be effective for some patients with fibromyalgia, but the overall differences between the treated group and the placebo group were neither clinically nor statistically significant.

**orofacial pain:** Heir (1997) and Bailey (1997) stress that pain problems associated with the orofacial region need to be evaluated thoroughly because the differential diagnosis is broad-ranging, including diseases such as Lyme disease and fibromyalgia.

**osteomalacia:** Reginato et al. (1999) point out that osteomalacia is usually neglected when compared with other metabolic bone diseases and may present with a variety of clinical and radiographic manifestations mimicking other musculoskeletal disorders, including fibromyalgia.

**osteoporosis:** Fibromyalgia is considered a risk factor and has been associated with osteoporosis. Early detection and implementation of appropriate nutritional supplementation (calcium/vitamin D), resistive and weight-bearing exercise, and specific bone mineral enhancing pharmacological therapy may be indicated in pre-, peri-, and postmenopausal subjects (Dessein and Stanwix, 2000; Swezey and Adams, 1999).

P **pain:** Fibromyalgia is associated with chronic widespread pain and decreased threshold for pain, features that are nonspecific (also present in other rheumatic conditions, such as rheumatoid arthritis), ill-defined and not well understood, and require careful evaluation for differential diagnosis (Alvarez-Lario et al., 1999; Atkins et al., 1995; Drewes, 1999; Ferguson and Ahles, 1998; Forseth et al., 1999; Friedman and Nelson, 1996; Gustafsson and Gaston-Johansson, 1996; Henriksson et al., 1996; MacFarlane et al., 1996; MacFarlane, 1999; Mountz et al., 1998; Nicassio et al., 1995; Reilly, 1999; Rubio Montanes et al., 1995; Smythe et al., 1997; Turk and Okifuji, 1997; Weigent et al., 1998; White and Harth, 1999; Zetterberg, 1996). Persistent pain in fibromyalgia is often difficult to understand and to treat, maybe because it is partially or wholly of nonnociceptive afferent origin (Bassoe, 1997; Bendtsen et al., 1997; Bengtsson and Henriksson, 1996; Houvenagel, 1999; Kosek et al., 1996; Kramis et al., 1996; Lidbeck, 1999; Lorenz et al., 1996; Sartin, 2000; Sorensen et al., 1998). Nonnociceptive pain is often an important component of pain associated with peripheral and central neuropathy, fibromyalgia, trauma-induced pain, idiopathic low back pain, and chronic regional pain syndrome. Nonnociceptive pain is often dependent upon central sensitization induced by prior or ongoing nociception. Chronic pain often differs from acute pain. The correlation between tissue pathology and the perceived severity of the chronic pain experience is poor or even absent. Furthermore, the sharp spatial localization of acute pain is not a feature of chronic pain; chronic pain is more diffuse and often spreads to areas beyond the original site. Also of importance: chronic pain seldom responds to the therapeutic measures that are successful in treating acute pain. Physicians who are unaware of these differences may label the patient with chronic pain as being neurotic or even a malingerer (Bennett, 1999).

Morris et al. (1998) used capsaicin-induced secondary hyperalgesia as a marker of abnormal nociceptive processing in fibromyalgia patients (Arner et al., 1998) and found enhanced sensitivity of nociceptive neurons at a spinal level, thereby supporting the concept of a generalized disturbance of pain modulation in this disorder (Bradley et al., 1997). Lautenbacher and Rollman (1997) also found that fibromyalgia patients had significantly lower heat pain thresholds than healthy subjects, but similar electrical detection and pain thresholds. Although repeatedly applied electrical stimuli resulted in a degree of perceptual adaptation that was similar between the two groups, concurrent tonic thermal stimuli, at both painful and nonpainful levels, significantly increased the electrical pain threshold in the healthy subjects but not in the fibromyalgia patients.

Integration of nociceptive signaling comprises peripheral, spinal, and supraspinal sites of the nervous system, and various excitatory or inhibitory neurotransmitter and modulator systems participate in pain processing and modulation (Schadrack and Zieglgansberger, 1998). The role of different neuroendocrine mediators in pain associated with fibromyalgia has been the subject of intense study (Russell, 1998; Weigent et al., 1998). For instance, Ernberg et al. (2000) reported that injection of serotonin (5HT) into the masseter muscle leads to pain and allodynia/hyperalgesia in healthy female controls but not in female fibromyalgia patients. Pain perception, therefore, appears to be differentially modulated in fibromyalgia patients (Bradley et al., 1997). In this respect, Kosek and Hansson (1997) found that although fibromyalgia patients did not differ from healthy controls in their response to vibratory stimulation in the forearm, no modulation of pressure pain was induced by heterotopic noxious conditioning stimulation, as opposed to controls, suggesting a dysfunction in systems subserving diffuse noxious inhibitory controls. Sorensen et al. (1997) also reported that different patient subgroups may show abnormalities in different pain-processing mechanisms.

Pain in fibromyalgia has several consequences. Agargun et al. (1999) reported that there is a negative correlation between pain and sleep disturbance: increased pain sensitivity is associated with greater sleep disturbance. Also, poor sleep results in increased pain severity and increased pain attention (Affleck et al., 1996).

**pain syndromes:** Pain syndromes can be divided anatomically into those that cause generalized pain, such as fibromyalgia syndrome and myofascial pain syndromes, and those that are confined to one regional anatomical area (Carette, 1996). The latter group comprise those of the neck, shoulder, elbow, wrist/hand, hip, knee, and ankle/foot (Linaker et al., 1999). Diffuse pain syndromes, such as fibromyalgia, are more common in women and also some, such as fibromyalgia and polymyalgia rheumatica, in older persons (Gowin, 2000). Fibromyalgia also may be a secondary phenomenon associated with some of the other diffuse pain syndromes, such as those of neoplastic or endocrinological etiology.

Several chronic pain syndromes may mimic fibromyalgia by (1) the occurrence of widespread pain, (2) the chronicity of complaints, (3) the preponderance of females in some of these, and (4) the lack of objective data to be derived from imaging techniques and laboratory tests (Menninger, 1998). Differential diagnosis requires examination of the locomotor system under biomechanical auspices both at rest and during movement to diagnose hyper- and hypomobility syndromes; treatment of these conditions is guided by principles to improve biomechanical function. In addition, the skin needs to be examined to detect panniculosis (also called cellulitis), which may be mixed with fibromyalgia due to its preferential occurrence in peri- or postmenopausal women (Menninger, 1998). Vertebral fractures and fibromyalgia, although very different and unrelated clinical conditions, are common pain conditions that can, at times, be difficult to diagnose and manage (Hall, 1999). Distinction between fibromyalgia and other chronic pain syndromes is also relevant in terms of prognosis, as illustrated by a study by MacFarlane et al. (1996), which found that although chronic widespread pain in the community has a generally good prognosis, those with additional symptoms associated with fibromyalgia were more likely still to have chronic widespread pain two years later.

**pentazocine-induced fibrous myopathy:** A case report by Sinsawaiwong et al. (1998) on a forty-seven-year-old woman who had a four-year history of intramuscular pentazocine injections in the lower extremities and who developed gradual stiffness and weakness of the lower extremities illustrates that caution in long-term usage and early recognition of pentazocine toxicity as a neuromuscular complication are important in order to prevent irreversible drug-induced fibrous myopathy and localized neuropathy. The latter condition should also be differentiated from fibromyalgia.

**Persian Gulf War syndrome:** Since the Persian Gulf War ended in 1991, veterans have reported an increased prevalence, as compared to contemporary military personnel who were not deployed, of diverse, unexplained symptoms, including some consistent with chronic fatigue syndrome, fibromyalgia, and multiple chemical sensitivity (Alloway et al., 1998; Hodgson and Kipen, 1999; Nicolson and Nicolson, 1998; "Self-Reported Illness and Health Status Among Gulf War Veterans: A Population-Based Study," 1997). Although some veterans have wondered if their development of systemic lupus erythematosus, amyotrophic lateral sclerosis, or fibromyalgia might be related to Gulf War service, an examination by Smith et al. (2000) of hospitalizations of regular, active-duty service personnel deployed to the Persian Gulf War ($n$ = 551,841) compared with nondeployed Gulf War-era service personnel ($n$ = 1,478,704) did not support Gulf War service and disease associations. Other controlled epidemiological studies in Gulf War veterans and controls describe significant excesses of symptoms that were not clearly associated with pathologic disease (Hodgson and Kipen, 1999).

Grady et al. (1998) reported that of 250 Gulf War veterans evaluated, 139 (56 percent) were referred for rheumatology consultation, which was the most common elective subspecialty referral. Of the patients evaluated, 82 (59 percent) had soft tissue syndromes, 19 (14 percent) had rheumatic disease, and 38 (27 percent) had no rheumatic disease. The most common soft tissue syndromes were patellofemoral syndrome (33 patients [24 percent]), mechanical low back pain (23 patients [17 percent]), and fibromyalgia (22 patients [16 percent]). Grady et al. (1998) concluded that the rheumatic manifestations in Gulf War veterans are similar to symptoms and diagnoses described in previous wars and are not unique to active-duty soldiers. After analyzing the rheumatic manifestations of 145 Persian Gulf War veterans, Escalante and Fischbach (1998) found that although the most common diagnosis was fibromyalgia (33.8 percent), followed by various soft tissue problems (17.2 percent), clinical or radiographic osteoarthritis (11.0 percent), and nonspecific arthralgias (9.6 percent), no specific rheumatic diagnosis is characteristic of Gulf War veterans with unexplained illness. However, pain is common and widespread in these patients, and their health-related quality of life is poor. Further research is necessary to determine the cause of the symptoms of veterans of the Gulf War.

**phenobarbital:** A case report by Goldman and Krings (1995) illustrates fibromyalgia induced by the anticonvulsant phenobarbital in a female swimming instructor who was seen with chronic bilateral shoulder pain and loss of range of motion. The patient, who was taking medication for tonic/clonic seizures, recalled that her symptoms began after her anticonvulsant medication was switched from hydantoin sodium to phenobarbital.

**phosphate diabetes:** Based on measurements of phosphate reabsorption by the proximal renal tubule, phosphate clearance, and renal threshold phosphate concentration, nine out of eighty-seven CFS patients in one study also fulfilled the diagnostic criteria for phosphate diabetes (phosphate depletion due to abnormal renal reabsorption of phosphate by the proximal tubule) (De Lorenzo et al., 1998). De Lorenzo and colleagues concluded that phosphate diabetes should be considered in the differential diagnosis of CFS. Laroche and Tack (1999) also pointed out that hypophosphoremia secondary to moderate idiopathic phosphate diabetes should be included in the differential diagnosis of primary fibromyalgia.

**physical therapy:** Physical therapy for fibromyalgia is aimed at disease consequences such as pain, fatigue, deconditioning, muscle weakness, sleep disturbances, and other disease consequences (Meng-shoel, 1997). A review by Offenbacher and Stucki (2000) concluded that, based on evidence from randomized controlled trials, cardiovascular fitness training significantly improves cardiovascular fitness, both subjective and objective measures of pain, as well as subjective energy and work capacity, and physical and social activities. Moreover, based on anecdotal evidence of small observational studies, physiotherapy may reduce overloading of the muscle system, improve postural fatigue and positioning, and condition weak muscles.

**platelet alpha-2-adrenoreceptors:** In the search for disease markers, Maes et al. (1999) found that fibromyalgia, particularly in the early phase of illness, is accompanied by lowered affinity of platelet alpha-2-adrenoreceptors. Further studies are needed to assess the usefulness of the latter observation.

**polymyalgia rheumatica:** Polymyalgia rheumatica (PMR) is a disease of unknown etiology characterized by severe myalgia and stiffness in shoulder girdle and pelvic girdle muscles and by normal serum creatine kinase levels. Marked elevation of erythrocyte sedimentation rate, acute onset within two weeks, and appearance in the aged are also additional characteristics of PMR. Ten to 50 percent of PMR patients have a concomitant temporal arteritis (giant cell arteritis). For the differential diagnoses of PMR, rheumatoid arthritis, polymyositis, fibromyalgia, malignancies, infections, and depression should be considered (Nishikai, 1999) (*see also* AGING AND GERIATRICS).

**postcardiac injury rheumatism:** Another disorder listed in the differential diagnosis for fibromyalgia is postcardiac injury rheumatism (PIR) (Mukhopadhyay et al., 1995). In a study by Mukhopadhyay et al. (1995), out of the 249 patients who survived cardiac surgery, twenty (8 percent) and twenty-two (9 percent) patients had early and late PIR, respectively. Earlier onset (within two weeks of surgery), milder articular involvement, absence of constitutional features and laboratory abnormalities, and good response to analgesics were characteristics of early PIR. In contrast, late PIR, which occurred between the third and fourteenth week after surgery, was associated with more marked articular involvement along with systemic and laboratory abnormalities and required longer analgesic therapy, steroid support, or prolonged physiotherapy in different combinations.

**post-Lyme disease syndrome:** Despite antibiotic treatment, a sequel of Lyme disease (or Lyme borreliosis) may be a post-Lyme disease syndrome characterized by persistent arthralgia, fatigue, and neuro-cognitive impairment that is probably induced by Lyme disease. Bujak et al. (1996) found that of twenty-three patients with post-Lyme disease syndrome, seven (30 percent) had fibromyalgia, three (13 percent) had chronic fatigue syndrome, and ten (43 percent) had similar but milder symptoms but did not meet the criteria for either. Late Lyme disease or post-Lyme disease syndrome must be distin-guished by clinical characteristics from fibromyalgia (the most com-mon source of misdiagnosis in several studies) (Berman and Wenglin, 1995; Ellenbogen, 1997; Rahn and Felz, 1998). A case can be defined as borreliosis only if either the typical erythema migrans is reliably identified by a physician or if a characteristic late manifestation of Lyme disease is accompanied by unequivocal serological and/or bac-teriological evidence of *Borrelia burgdorferi* infection (Frey et al., 1995, 1998; Graninger, 1996; Nadelman et al., 1999; Sigal, 1995). Within the musculoskeletal system, the only reliable characteristic symptom is true synovitis, as defined by the palpable swelling of a joint. Mere joint pain or the subjective pain syndrome of fibromyal-gia do not constitute a defining symptom for borreliosis (Graninger, 1996). Fallon et al. (1999) reported increased Fibromyalgia Impact Questionnaire total score, muscle pain, and joint pain in fibromyalgia patients as compared to post-Lyme disease syndrome patients.

**postpolio syndrome:** Fibromyalgia may mimic some of the symp-toms of postpoliomyelitis syndrome, a disorder characterized by new weakness, fatigue, and pain decades after paralytic poliomyelitis (Trojan and Cashman, 1995). Trojan and Cashman (1995) found that ten (10.5 percent) of ninety-five postpolio patients met the criteria for fibromyalgia, and another ten patients (10.5 percent) had borderline fibromyalgia. Postpolio syndrome patients with fibromyalgia were more likely than patients without fibromyalgia to be female (80 percent versus 40 percent) and to complain of generalized fatigue (100 per-cent versus 71 percent) but were not distinguishable in terms of age at presentation to clinic, age at polio, length of time since polio, physical activity, weakness at polio, motor strength scores on examination, and presence of new weakness, muscle fatigue, or joint pain. Approximately 50 percent of postpolio syndrome patients in both the fibromyalgia and borderline fibromyalgia groups responded to low-dose, nighttime amitriptyline therapy.

**post-traumatic stress disorder:** Traumatic events can result in a set of symptoms including nightmares, recurrent and intrusive recollections, avoidance of thoughts or activities associated with the traumatic event, and symptoms of increased arousal such as insomnia and hypervigilance. These post-traumatic stress disorder (PTSD)-like symptoms are frequently observed in persons with chronic pain syndromes. Approximately 56 percent of a sample of ninety-three fibromyalgia patients studied by Sherman et al. (2000) reported clinically significant levels of PTSD-like symptoms (PTSD+). The PTSD+ patients reported significantly greater levels of pain, emotional distress, life interference, and disability than did the patients without clinically significant levels of PTSD-like symptoms (PTSD–). Over 85 percent of the PTSD+ patients, compared with 50 percent of the PTSD– patients, demonstrated significant disability. Based on response to the Multidimensional Pain Inventory, a significantly lower percentage of PTSD+ patients were classified as adaptive copers (15 percent) compared with the PTSD– group (48.2 percent) (Sherman et al., 2000). Amir et al. (1997) also documented that PTSD subjects suffering from fibromyalgia were more tender and reported more pain, lower quality of life, and higher functional impairment, and suffered more psychological distress than the PTSD patients without fibromyalgia. Therefore, clinicians should assess the presence of these symptoms, as the failure to attend to them in treatment may impede successful outcomes.

**propyl endopeptidase:** Maes et al. (1998) found that fibromyalgia patients have significantly lower serum activities of prolyl endopeptidase (PEP) but normal activities of dipeptidyl peptidase IV (DPP IV). Serum PEP activity was negatively correlated with severity of pressure hyperalgesia and the nonsomatic, cognitive symptoms of the Hamilton Depression Rating Scale. Fibromyalgia patients with severe pressure hyperalgesia had significantly lower PEP activity than normal controls and fibromyalgia patients with less severe hyperalgesia, observations that are consistent with a relationship between low PEP activity and abnormal pain perception. Fibromyalgia patients with severe nonsomatic depressive symptoms had significantly lower serum PEP activity than normal volunteers. Lower serum PEP activity may play a role in the biophysiology of fibromyalgia through diminished inactivation of algesic and depression-related peptides (Maes et al., 1998).

**prostaglandin D synthase:** Prostaglandin D synthase (PGD synthase) or beta-trace protein is a major constituent of human cerebrospinal fluid (CSF), representing 3 percent of the total CSF protein. Normally, PGD synthase levels in CSF are approximately thirty-fivefold higher than those of serum, with a median concentration of 11,299 µg/L. Melegos et al. (1997) found no statistical difference between PGD synthase concentrations in the CSF or the serum of patients with different diseases, such as multiple sclerosis, HIV/AIDS-related neuropathies, viral meningitis, and fibromyalgia. Therefore, PGD synthase measurement has no clinical utility in diagnosing neurological disorders in adulthood.

**protein peroxidation:** Eisinger et al. (1996) demonstrated increased protein peroxidation (elevated protein carbonyls) in twenty-five fibromyalgia patients. The relevance of this observation needs further substantiation.

**psychiatry:** Patients with chronic widespread pain (CWP) have been reported to have a greater prevalence of mental disorders and somatization than that found in the general population (Avina-Zubieta et al., 1997; Ben-Zion et al., 1996; Ruderman and Golden, 1996). A population-based case-control study by Benjamin et al. (2000) of 710 subjects, although unable to demonstrate a cause-and-effect relationship, showed that 16.9 percent of those with CWP were estimated to have a psychiatric diagnosis, suggesting that these disorders should be identified and treated. Offenbaecher et al. (1998) found clinically relevant depression in 27 percent of 304 fibromyalgia patients studied. Meyer-Lindenberg and Gallhofer (1998) proposed that the subgroup of fibromyalgia patients with depressive symptoms may be pragmatically classified as suffering from somatized depression, and Keel (1998) pointed out that fibromyalgia patients most often present with persistent somatoform pain disorder (ICD-10) and dysthymia than with major psychiatric disorders. In a multicenter study of seventy-three individuals, Epstein et al. (1999) found that fibromyalgia patients exhibited high levels of some lifetime or current psychiatric disorders (mainly depression, 22 percent, and panic disorders, 7 percent) and significant current psychological distress. A study by Aaron et al. (1996) yielded similar results. Current anxiety level appears to be an important correlate of functional impairment in fibromyalgia patients (Epstein et al., 1999). Repeated traumatic experiences during childhood and as adults can be discovered in many cases, which helps in understanding some of the difficulties met in psychotherapy with fibromyalgia patients (Keel, 1998).

Antidepressant treatment is generally beneficial in fibromyalgia, but improvement in symptomatology does not necessarily correlate with treatment of comorbid psychiatric conditions (Dunne and Dunne, 1995; Gruber et al., 1996; Hudson and Pope, 1996) (*see also* ANTIDE-PRESSANTS), an observation that curtails those who favor a psychiatric etiology of diffuse pain syndromes. In this respect, a study by Katz and Kravitz (1996) suggests that the tendency toward depression in fibromyalgia patients may be a manifestation of a familial depressive spectrum disorder (alcoholism and/or depression in family members), not simply a "reactive" depression secondary to the pain and other symptoms.

**psychosocial factors:** In fibromyalgia, psychosocial factors are relevant at different levels (predisposing, triggering, and stabilizing/ "chronifying" factors) (Affleck et al., 1998; Anderberg, 1999; Eich et al., 2000; Rosenfeld and Walco, 1997; Walker et al., 1997). Hallberg and Carlsson (1998) found that individuals with insecure attachment styles are overrepresented among patients with chronic pain. Wolfe and Hawley (1998) pointed out that psychosocial distress and psychological abnormality occurs frequently in fibromyalgia patients (Jamison, 1999a,b) (*see* AFFECTIVE DISTRESS AND ANXIETY). Patterns of decreased levels of education and increased rates of divorce, obesity, and smoking have been noted in clinical and epidemiological studies (Neumann and Buskila, 1998). Links to physical and sexual abuse have been noted as well (*see* ABUSE). Major depression as well as increased rates of depression, anxiety, and somatization are also commonly found in fibromyalgia (*see* DEPRESSION, PSYCHIA-

TRY). Turk et al. (1998) suggest that customizing fibromyalgia treatment based on patients' psychosocial needs will lead to enhanced treatment efficacy.

**quality of life:** Quality of life is significantly affected in patients with rheumatic diseases, such as fibromyalgia, rheumatoid arthritis, and Sjogren's syndrome (Buskila et al., 1997; Ruiz Moral et al., 1997; Strombeck et al., 2000). Comorbid conditions such as anxiety and depression further affect quality of life (Kurtze et al., 1999). Schlenk et al. (1998) found that fibromyalgia patients had comparable quality-of-life scores to patients with chronic obstructive pulmonary disease, AIDS, or urinary incontinence, and worse than patients with prostate cancer or hyperlipidemia. Wolfe and Hawley (1997) found that fibromyalgia patients have lower quality-of-life scores compared to patients with rheumatoid arthritis or osteoarthritis. Patients' perceptions and coping styles also determine quality of life (Soderberg et al., 1997). Neumann and Buskila (1997) reported that the quality of life and physical functioning of the relatives of fibromyalgia patients were impaired, especially for female relatives and those with undiagnosed fibromyalgia, a finding that may be attributed to the psychological distress in families of fibromyalgia patients and to the high prevalence (25 percent) of undiagnosed fibromyalgia among relatives.

**Raynaud's phenomenon:** Raynaud's phenomenon has also been reported among patients with fibromyalgia (Grassi et al., 1998).

**rehabilitation:** After an extensive review of the literature, Karjalainen et al. (2000) concluded that there appears to be little scientific evidence for the effectiveness of multidisciplinary rehabilitation for musculoskeletal disorders, including fibromyalgia. However, multidisciplinary rehabilitation is a commonly used intervention for chronic musculoskeletal disorders (Epifanov and Epifanov, 2000), which cause much personal suffering and substantial economic loss to the society (Berg et al., 1998). Buckelew et al. (1996)

found that higher levels of self-efficacy are associated with better outcome and may mediate the effectiveness of rehabilitation-based treatment programs for fibromyalgia. There is a need for high quality trials in this field.

**rhinitis:** Rhinitis symptoms are present in approximately 70 percent of subjects with fibromyalgia and chronic fatigue syndrome (FM/CFS). Because only 35 percent to 50 percent have positive allergy skin tests, nonallergic mechanisms may also play a role. Baraniuk et al. (1998) found no differences in the basal secretion of markers of vascular permeability, submucosal gland serous cell secretion, and eosinophil and neutrophil degranulation in nonallergic FM/CFS subjects. Irritant rhinitis has been associated with FM/CFS (Baraniuk et al., 2000).

**ritanserin:** Ritanserin is a long-acting serotonin (5-hydroxytryptamine) 2 (5-HT2)-receptor blocker. In a sixteen-week study of fifty-one female fibromyalgia patients, Olin et al. (1998) found that, at the end of the study, there was an improvement in feeling refreshed in the morning in the ritanserin-treated group and that headache was also significantly improved compared with the placebo group. There was no difference in pain, fatigue, sleep, morning stiffness, anxiety, and tender point counts in the ritanserin and placebo groups. Fifty-one percent of the fifty-one patients had at least one of the three antibodies to 5-HT, Gm1, and phospholipids. The incidence and activity of these antibodies were not influenced by ritanserin or placebo. The observation that ritanserin has only a small effect on clinical symptoms indicates that disturbances in serotonin metabolism or uptake may be only one factor in the pathogenesis of the disease.

**rubella vaccines:** The National Vaccine Injury Compensation Program and the United States Court of Federal Claims have accepted a causal relationship between currently used rubella vaccine in the United States and some chronic arthropathy with an onset between one week and six weeks after vaccine administration. Fibromyalgia was reported in four out of seventy-two subjects with chronic arthropathy developing between one week and six weeks after the rubella vaccination, and in eleven out of fifty-two individuals in whom chronic arthropathy developed in less than one week or greater than six weeks postvaccination (Weibel and Benor, 1996).

**S-adenosyl-L-methionine:** A short-term crossover study by Volkmann et al. (1997) on thirty-four fibromyalgia patients showed no effect of intravenous administration of 600 mg for ten days of S-adenosyl-L-methionine (SAMe). Tavoni et al. (1998) also failed to demonstrate statistically significant effects of SAMe on secondary fibromyalgia.

**saliva:** Because of accessibility, measurement of neuropeptides in human saliva could provide a valuable tool for study of patients with chronic painful disorders, such as rheumatoid arthritis, osteoarthritis, and fibromyalgia (Fischer et al., 1998).

**sarcoid arthritis:** Gran and Bohmer (1996) reported the development of secondary fibromyalgia in two patients with sarcoid arthritis. Although acute sarcoid arthritis is usually a self-limiting joint disease, recurrences may occasionally occur and some cases develop chronic sarcoidosis of the lungs.

**scleritis:** Fan and Florakis (1996) presented a case report of a patient with scleritis and fibromyalgia and proposed that additional cases might suggest that fibromyalgia be added to the list of etiologies of scleritis.

**selective serotonin reuptake inhibitors (fluoxetine, citalopram):** Several authors have recommended the use of selective serotonin reuptake inhibitors (SSRIs), such as fluoxetine (Prozac), in the management of chronic pain and fibromyalgia (Anderbeg et al., 2000; Chambliss, 1998; Nerhood, 1998). However, Norregaard et al. (1995) failed to find a positive effect for citalopram in fibromyalgia, and Smith (1998) suggests that there is little evidence for the replacement of tricyclic antidepressants with SSRIs in pain management. Based on a review of the literature, Jung et al. (1997) concluded that it is unclear whether SSRIs are beneficial for migraine headaches, tension headaches, diabetic neuropathy, or fibromyalgia and recommended that it may be reasonable to reserve SSRIs for those who fail to respond to other medications or who are intolerant of their side effects. In a four-week trial of 20 mg fluoxetine and 25 mg of amitriptyline, alone or in combination, Goldenberg et al. (1996) found that both medications are effective treatments for fibromyalgia (pain, well-being, sleep), and they work better in combination than either medication alone.

**selenium:** Reinhard et al. (1998) reported decreased serum concentrations of selenium among sixty-eight fibromyalgia patients in Germany, although there was overlap in the range of concentrations as compared to ninety-seven controls.

**self-esteem:** Johnson et al. (1997) in a study of thirty-six depressed fibromyalgia patients found that they had a high need to gain self-esteem through competence and others' approval. This was combined with a low basic sense of self-esteem. Nondepressed fibromyalgia patients did not display this self-esteem pattern. Based on the latter observations, Johnson et al. (1997) suggest that an emphatic competence-dependent self-esteem is one vulnerability factor that, in proper genetic and environmental conditions, increases susceptibility to fibromyalgia and depression.

**serotonin:** Ernberg, Hedenberg-Magnusson, Alstergren, and Kopp, (1999) found that serotonin is present in the human masseter muscle both immediately following puncture and also in a subsequent steady state and that it is associated with pain and allodynia. The origin of the serotonin seems to be partly the blood, but peripheral release also occurs (Sprott et al., 1998). Allodynia of orofacial muscles in patients with temporomandibular disorder is significantly related to serotonin concentration (Ernberg, Hedenberg-Magnusson, Alstergren, Lundeberg, et al., 1999). Ernberg et al. (1998) also found that there is a reduction of the ratio between initial serotonin and steady state level in the painful masseter muscle after intramuscular glucocorticoid administration to fibromyalgia patients, a reduction not present in localized myalgia patients. Serotonin seems to be involved in the modulation of local muscle microcirculation in fibromyalgia patients and in hyperalgesia in localized myalgia patients (Ernberg et al., 1998; Wolfe et al., 1997). A defect in serotonergic analgesia and a hyperalgesic state are proposed as features common to headache and fibromyalgia

(Nicolodi et al., 1998). The benefit to both migraine and fibromyalgia from inhibiting ionotropic N-methyl-D-aspartate receptor activity implies that redundant hyperalgesia-related neuroplastic changes are crucial for severe or chronic migraine and primary fibromyalgia (Nicolodi et al., 1998). Serotonin substrate supplementation, via L-tryptophan or 5-hydroxytryptophan, has been shown to improve symptoms of depression, anxiety, insomnia, and somatic pains in a variety of fibromyalgia patient cohorts (Juhl, 1998).

**serotonin 3-receptor antagonists (Tropisetron, Ondansetron):** Serotonin (5-HT) 3-receptor antagonists are potent and highly selective competitive inhibitors of the 5-HT3-receptor with negligible affinity for other receptors. They are rapidly absorbed and penetrate the blood-brain barrier easily (Wolf, 2000). 5-HT3-receptor antagonists do not modify any aspect of normal behavior in animals or induce remarkable changes of physiological functions in healthy subjects. They are well tolerated over wide dose ranges; the most common side effects in clinical use are headache and obstipation. Clinical efficacy was first established in chemotherapy-induced emesis, and other established indications are radiotherapy-induced and postoperative emesis. Antiemetic efficacy results from a simultaneous action at peripheral and central 5-HT3-receptors. Other peripheral actions include reduction of secretion and diarrhea caused by increased intestinal serotonin content (e.g., in carcinoid syndrome), a limited antiarrhythmic activity and a reduction of experimentally induced pain. CNS effects comprise anxiolysis, attenuation of age-associated memory impairment, reduction of alcohol consumption in moderate alcohol abuse, and an antipsychotic effect in patients with Parkinson psychosis. In migraine, 5-HT3-receptor antagonists show moderate efficacy, as well. Repeatedly demonstrated efficacy of 5-HT3-receptor antagonists in patients suffering from fibromyalgia raises the question for the mechanism of action involved. Ligand binding at the 5-HT3-receptor causes manifold effects on other neurotransmitter and neuropeptide systems. In particular, 5-HT3-receptor antagonists diminish serotonin-induced release of substance P from C-fibers and prevent unmasking of NK2-receptors in the presence of serotonin (Wolf, 2000). The effect of the 5-HT3-receptor antagonists is probable primarily to limit the release of substance P, which acts as a pain and inflammatory mediator, and is itself released by the neurogenic inflammation that occurs after the binding of serotonin to its corresponding receptor (Stratz and Muller, 2000a,b). Intraarticular injection of the 5-HT3-receptor antagonist, tropisetron, results in improvement on different types of local rheumatic pain and inflammatory processes (Stratz and Muller, 2000a,b). Intravenous administration of 2 mg of tropisetron or oral administration of 5 mg daily are well tolerated and result in reduction of pain associated with fibromyalgia (Farber et al., 2000; Haus et al., 2000; Muller and Stratz, 2000; Papadopoulos et al., 2000; Samborski et al., 1996) and improvement of comorbid depression (Haus et al., 2000). However, there are no clear biochemical markers (including serum concentrations of serotonin, somatomedin C, oxytocin, calcitonin-gene-related peptide, calcitonin, and cholecystokinin) associated with the effect of tropisetron in fibromyalgia (Hocherl et al., 2000; Stratz and Muller, 2000a). Hrycaj et al. (1996) found that the 5-HT3-receptor antagonist ondansetron also appears to be effective in about 50 percent of fibromyalgia patients.

**serotonin receptor gene:** The T102 allele of the *serotonin2A-receptor* gene might be involved in the complex circuits of nociception. Although a study of 168 fibromyalgia patients failed to evince that the T102C polymorphism is directly involved in the etiology of fibromyalgia, it might be in linkage dysequilibrium with the true functional variant, which has to be unraveled (Bondy et al., 1999).

**serotonin transporter gene:** A higher frequency of the S/S genotype of the serotonin transporter gene (5-HTT) was found among sixty-two fibromyalgia patients compared with 110 healthy controls (31 percent versus 16 percent). The S/S subgroup exhibited higher mean levels of depression and psychological distress. These results support the notion of altered serotonin metabolism in at least a subgroup of fibromyalgia patients (Offenbaecher et al., 1999).

**serum nucleotide pyrophosphohydrolase:** Another possible marker tested for fibromyalgia was not specific per the study by Cardenal et al. (1998), who found elevated levels of serum nucleotide pyrophosphohydrolase in patients with degenerative arthritis whether or not calcium pyrophosphate crystals were present, in patients with either scleroderma or fibromyalgia, and in patients receiving hemodialysis therapy or taking cyclosporine.

**Sjogren's syndrome:** Sjogren's syndrome, the second most common autoimmune rheumatic disease, refers to keratoconjunctivitis sicca and xerostomia resulting from immune lymphocytes that infiltrate the lacrimal and salivary glands (Fox et al., 2000). Sjogren's syndrome is included in the differential for the diagnosis for fibromyalgia, and the distinction between fibromyalgia patients with low titer antinuclear antibodies and primary Sjogren's syndrome remains difficult (Fox, 1997; Fox et al., 1998). Giles and Isenberg (2000) reported that fibromyalgia was present in nine out of seventy-four (12 percent) patients with primary Sjogren's syndrome compared with eleven of 216 (5 percent) lupus patients and none of secondary Sjogren's syndrome patients. Giles and Isenberg (2000) also reported that fatigue in patients with primary or secondary Sjogren's syndrome is not due to the coexistence of fibromyalgia in most cases. Dohrenbusch et al. (1996) found a higher prevalence of fibromyalgia in Sjogren's syndrome (44 percent among primary and 5 percent among secondary Sjogren's syndrome patients).

**skinache syndrome:** Chronic pain of unknown etiology, and characterized by cutaneous trigger points, has been coined skinache syndrome (Bassoe, 1995). In contrast to fibromyalgia, skinache syndrome has a simple and effective cure: subcutaneous injection of lidocaine.

**sleep:** Nonrestorative sleep is a prominent feature of fibromyalgia; unrefreshing sleep occurs in 76 to 90 percent of fibromyalgia patients compared with 10 to 30 percent of controls (Campbell et al., 1983; Green, 1999; Hemmeter et al., 1995; Hench, 1996; Kempenaers et al., 1994; Lugaresi et al., 1981; Moldofsky, 1989; Moldofsky et al., 1975; Reilly and Littlejohn, 1993; Roizenblatt et al., 2001; Schaefer, 1995; Smythe, 1995; Smythe and Moldofsky, 1977; Wolfe and Cathey, 1983; Wolfe et al., 1990; Yunus et al., 1981). Fibromyalgia patients report early morning awakenings, awakening feeling tired or unrefreshed, insomnia, as well as mood and cognitive disturbances; they may also experience primary sleep disorders, including sleep apnea (Harding, 1998). Sleep disturbances contribute to overnight pain and stiffness exacerbation and increased pain sensitivity in fibromyalgia and other chronic musculoskeletal pain conditions (Affleck et al., 1996; Agargun et al., 1999; Croft et al., 1994; Greenberg et al., 1995; Hemmeter et al., 1995; Hirsch et al., 1994; Kryeger,

1995; Kryger and Shapiro, 1992; Leigh et al., 1998; Mahowald et al., 1989; Moldofsky and Scarisbrick, 1976; Older et al., 1998; Roizenblatt et al., 1997; Scharf et al., 1998; Walsh et al., 1994; Wittig et al., 1982), and poor sleep is associated with psychological distress and cognitive dysfunction (Affleck et al., 1996; Côte and Moldofsky, 1997; Hansotia, 1996; Hyyppa and Kronholm, 1995; Paiva et al., 1995; Phillips and Cousins, 1986; Pilowski et al., 1985; Shaver et al., 1997).

Among the disruptions in sleep architecture in fibromyalgia patients, there is evidence for prolonged sleep latencies (Branco et al., 1994; Horne and Shackeel, 1991), low sleep efficiency (Touchon et al., 1988; Wittig et al., 1982), an increased amount of stage 1 non–rapid eye movement (non-REM) sleep (Anch et al., 1991; Branco et al., 1994; Harding, 1998; Moldofsky et al., 1975; Sergi et al., 1999; Shaver et al., 1997), the presence of alpha electroencephalographic activity during non-REM sleep (Branco et al., 1994; Drewes, Gade, et al., 1995; Drewes, Nielsen, et al., 1995; Flanigan et al., 1995; Harding, 1998; MacFarlane et al., 1996; Moldofsky et al., 1975; Perlis et al., 1997; Roizenblatt et al., 1997, 2001; Ware et al., 1986), a reduction in slow-wave sleep (Branco et al. 1994; Drewes et al., 1995, 1996; Horne and Shackeel, 1991; Touchon et al., 1988) and in REM percentages (Branco et al., 1994), an increased number of arousals (Branco et al., 1994; Clauw et al., 1994; Harding, 1998; Horne and Shackeel, 1991; Molony et al., 1986; Shaver et al., 1997; Staedt et al., 1993; Touchon et al., 1988), periodic breathing (Sergi et al., 1999) and arterial oxygen desaturations (Alvarez-Lario et al., 1996), and restless leg movements (Atkinson et al., 1988; Wittig et al., 1982; Yunus and Aldag, 1996).

Lentz et al. (1999) reported that disruption of slow-wave sleep in healthy volunteers, without reducing total sleep or sleep efficiency, for several consecutive nights is associated with decreased pain threshold, increased discomfort, fatigue, and the inflammatory flare response in skin. Also, deep pain induced during sleep in normal controls causes the alpha frequency rhythm, termed alpha-delta sleep anomaly, which is seen in fibromyalgia patients and in normal controls during stage 4 sleep deprivation (Fischler et al., 1997; Harding, 1998). These results suggest that disrupted sleep is probably an important factor in the pathophysiology of symptoms in fibromyalgia.

The association between sleep disturbances and pain and other fibromyalgia symptoms has been challenged by several studies. Older et al. (1998) found that three nights of delta-wave sleep interruption caused no significant lowering of pain thresholds or serum insulin-like growth factor 1 (IGF-1) in healthy volunteers, thereby concluding that the low levels of IGF-1 seen in fibromyalgia patients may result from chronic rather than acute delta-wave sleep interruption, or may be dependent on factors other than disturbances of delta-wave sleep. Tishler et al. (1997) also reported that sleep abnormalities and fibromyalgia in primary Sjogren's syndrome patients are frequent and that their etiology might involve other mechanisms besides joint pain or sicca symptomatology. Donald et al. (1996) reported that although fibromyalgia was uncommon (2.7 percent) in patients with a primary complaint of disturbed sleep and, in particular, patients with sleep apnea, reduced physical activity was strongly associated with reported pain symptoms.

Harding (1998) recommends that before prescribing pharmacologic compounds aimed at modifying sleep, adequate pain control and sleep habits should be achieved; tricyclic antidepressants, trazodone, zopiclone, and selective serotonin reuptake inhibitors may be required (Touchon, 1995).

**smoking:** Ostensen and Schei (1997) reported that smoking was significantly more frequent for Norwegian women reporting fibromyalgia. Anxiety and depression in fibromyalgia was associated with higher consumption of cigarettes (Kurtze et al., 1998, 1999). Tobacco use may adversely affect fibromyalgia (Aaron and Buchwald, 2000; Jay, 2000).

**social networks:** In a cross-sectional, retrospective, case-control study of twenty-five female fibromyalgia patients, Bolwijn et al. (1996) found that, compared to twenty-five healthy controls, the social networks of fibromyalgia patients presented more linkages with intimate friends, family members, and health care providers.

**sphenopalatine blocks:** Although sphenopalatine blocks have been used to treat pain for more than eighty years, Janzen and Scudds (1997), in a double-blind placebo-controlled study on sixty-one patients (forty-two with fibromyalgia and nineteen with myofascial pain syndrome) failed to find support for this technique by showing no statistical differences between the lidocaine and the placebo groups.

**spinal tracts:** In the spinal cord, long descending pathways are known to exist which modulate pain sensations by either inhibiting or facilitating the discharges of spinal nociceptive neurons. Mense (1998, 2000) has proposed that a dysfunction of the descending inhibitory pathways could mimic, to a large extent, the pain of fibromyalgia. Dorsal descending systems are tonicly active and have a particularly strong inhibitory action on neurons that mediate pain from deep tissues, and an impairment of their function is likely to lead to spontaneous deep pain (because of an increased background activity in nociceptive neurons supplying deep tissues); tenderness of deep tissues (because of a lowered mechanical threshold of the same neurons); and hyperalgesia of deep tissues (because of increased neuronal responses to noxious stimuli).

***Staphylococcus* toxoid vaccine:** Several studies have shown a positive effect of *Staphylococcus* toxoid vaccine in patients with fibromyalgia and chronic fatigue syndrome (Andersson et al., 1998). For instance, in a placebo-controlled study of twenty-eight patients who fulfilled the criteria for both fibromyalgia and chronic fatigue syndrome, significant improvements in fatiguability and pain were seen. In a follow-up study of twenty-three patients, the vaccine treatment was continued for two to six years. Fifty percent were rehabilitated successfully and resumed half-time or full-time work (Andersson et al., 1998).

**substance P:** Substance P is a putative nociceptive transmitter. The finding of significantly high levels of substance P in the cerebrospinal fluid of fibromyalgia patients (Larson et al., 2000; Liu et al., 2000) supports the impact of this neurotransmitter on both nociceptive and antinociceptive mechanisms (Pongratz and Sievers, 2000). Substance P levels are also elevated in the serum of fibromyalgia patients (Sprott et al., 1998). Schwarz et al. (1999) documented a strong negative correlation between serum substance P and 5-hydroxyindolacetic acid (5-HIAA) as well as between substance P and tryptophan in fibromyalgia patients. High serum concentrations of 5-HIAA and tryptophan showed a significant relation to low pain scores. More-over, 5-HIAA was strongly related to good quality of sleep, while substance P was related to sleep disturbance (Schwarz et al., 1999). In contrast to fibromyalgia, Evengard et al. (1998) found normal levels of substance P in the cerebrospinal fluid of fifteen patients with chronic fatigue syndrome, an observation that supports the notion that fibromyalgia and chronic fatigue syndrome are different dis-orders despite overlapping symptomatology.

**Super Malic:** In a study of twenty-four fibromyalgia patients who were randomized to a fixed dose (3 tablets b.i.d.), placebo-controlled, four-week-course pilot trial, followed by a six-month, open-label, dose escalation (up to 6 tablets b.i.d.) trial, Russell et al. (1995) found that Super Malic, a proprietary tablet containing malic acid (200 mg) and magnesium (50 mg), is safe and may be beneficial in the treat-ment of fibromyalgia patients. Further studies are necessary.

**surgeries:** ter Borg et al. (1999) found no differences in the fre-quency of abdominal surgery between eighty newly diagnosed fe-male fibromyalgia and forty-seven rheumatoid arthritis patients per-formed before the formal diagnosis. In the rheumatoid arthritis group more cholecystectomies were performed, probably due to the older age of these patients, whereas in the fibromyalgia group there were more hysterectomies (Wagener et al., 1997) and appendectomies than in the rheumatoid arthritis group.

**systemic lupus erythematosus:** Fibromyalgia and systemic lupus erythematosus (SLE) may be comorbid conditions (Bennett, 1997; Godfrey et al., 1998; Handa et al., 1998; Lopez-Osa et al., 1999; Romano, 1995, 1997; Wallace, 1995), and patients with SLE may be at increased risk to develop secondary fibromyalgia (Grafe et al., 1999). SLE is in the differential in the diagnosis of fibromyalgia (Calvo-Alen et al., 1995). Health-related quality of life is impaired both among women with fibromyalgia or SLE and with fibromyalgia patients reporting greater impairment along several dimensions (Da Costa et al., 2000). Bruce et al. (1999) documented that in an out-patient population of SLE patients (eighty-one studied), fatigue se-verity correlates with poor health status and a higher tender point count. Wang et al. (1998) also reported that fatigue in SLE patients is highly correlated with the presence of fibromyalgia and not with lupus disease activity. In patients with SLE, factors associated with quality of life and fibromyalgia seem to have a greater influence on the severity of reported fatigue than does the level of current disease activity (Abu-Shakra et al., 1999; Bruce et al., 1999; Gladman et al., 1997; Petri, 1995). Akkasilpa et al. (2000) found that SLE patients with fibromyalgic tender points are less likely to be good "copers."

Although fibomyalgia and SLE may coexist, Gladman et al. (2000) found that patients with inactive SLE demonstrate neurocognitive dysfunction that is not associated with comorbid fibromyalgia or with specific organ involvement or organ damage. Moreover, Taylor et al. (2000) reported that only a minority (10 percent of 216 assessed) of lupus patients with fatigue fulfill the American College of Rheumatology criteria for fibromyalgia. In one study, fibromyalgia symptomatology did not correlate with lupus severity (Grafe et al., 1999).

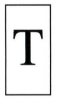 **temporomandibular disorder:** Patients with chronic fatigue syndrome, fibromyalgia, myofascial pain syndrome, and temporomandibular disorder (TMD) share many clinical illness features such as myalgia, fatigue, sleep disturbances, impairment in ability to perform activities of daily living as a consequence of these symptoms, and other comorbid conditions (such as irritable bowel syndrome, interstitial cystitis, and others) (Aaron et al., 2000). Fibromyalgia and myofascial pain syndrome are causes of TMD, and fibromyalgia patients often suffer from symptoms of TMD with the intensity of local pain correlating with that of general body pain (De Laat, 1997; Hedenberg-Magnusson et al., 1997, 1999; Pennacchio et al., 1998; Stohler, 1999). Conversely, patients with TMD and chronic facial pain may also manifest pain or increased pain sensitivity at remote sites outside of the head and neck region that may be secondary to impaired endogenous opioid systems (Kashima et al., 1999; Korszun et al., 1998; Wright et al., 1997) or to dysregulations in the hypothalamic-pituitary axis (Auvenshine, 1997). Miller et al. (1997) documented an unusual case of temporomandibular disorder in the presence of both fibromyalgia and Ehlers-Danlos syndrome. Plesh et al. (1996) point out that despite the overlap between fibromyalgia,

myofascial pain syndrome, and temporomandibular disorder, they are distinct clinical entities, and TMD patients show less evidence of distress than fibromyalgia patients.

**tender point pathophysiology:** Tender points are areas of tenderness occurring in muscles, muscle-tendon junctions, bursa, or fat pads. When tender points occur in a widespread manner, they are usually considered characteristic of fibromyalgia, and the presence of eleven out of eighteen tender points in defined locations in the body serves as part of the diagnostic criteria for fibromyalgia (Quimby et al., 1998; Sigal et al., 1998). Tender point examination is considered superior to dolorimetry (Wolfe, 1997). However, Tunks et al. (1995) reported that both dolorimetry and palpation are sufficiently reliable to discriminate control patients from patients with myofascial pain and fibromyalgia, but may not discriminate patients with myofascial pain from those with fibromyalgia.

McIntosh et al. (1998) reported that at least three subjects should be examined using three standards of reliability (80 percent, 85 percent, and 90 percent) before certification is granted to a health care professional. To minimize intrarater and interobserver variation in tender point examination, Smythe (1998) developed a training program that focused on learning to deliver 4 kg force as the pressure used in tender point examinations. Smythe (1998) recommends that these skills should be periodically refreshed to prevent drift into error. Okifuji et al. (1997) also developed a standardized tender point examination protocol (Manual Tender Point Survey [MTPS]) as a diagnostic procedure to evaluate the tender point criterion for fibromyalgia syndrome (sensitivity of 88.57 percent and specificity of 71.43 percent, comparable to the sensitivity and specificity of the 1990 multicenter study). Based on a study of eighty-four fibromyalgia patients, Wolfe (1998) points out that positive control points are a common feature (63 percent) in fibromyalgia and appear to be a marker for a generally low pain threshold rather than a disproportionate increase in severe symptoms or distress. Control point positivity should not be used to disqualify a diagnosis of fibromyalgia, and Wolfe (1998) suggests that their assessment should be abandoned in the manual tender point examination.

Tender point scores are related to generalized pain and pain behavior tendencies in fibromyalgia patients and do not independently reflect generalized psychological distress (Fassbender et al., 1997; Nicassio et al., 2000) as had been suggested by some authors (Croft et al., 1996; Mcbeth et al., 1999; Wolfe, 1997). In this respect, based on a study of 113 fibromyalgia patients, Jacobs et al. (1996) concluded that tender point scores and self-reported pain represent very different aspects of pain in fibromyalgia, the former being a more objective finding less prone to be affected by the patient's distress level. In a study of twenty fibromyalgia patients, Jeschonneck et al. (2000) found that vasoconstriction occurs in the skin above tender points in fibromyalgia patients, an observation that supports the hypothesis that fibromyalgia is related to local hypoxia in the skin above tender points. In another study of twenty fibromyalgia patients, Sprott et al. (2000) showed that acupuncture led to normalization of clinical parameters with improvement in microcirculation above tender points. The latter observations stand in contrast with an earlier study of sixteen fibromyalgia patients by Kosek et al. (1995), who found that pressure-induced pain sensibility in fibromyalgia patients is not most pronounced in muscle tissue and does not depend on increased skin sensibility.

Tender points and fibromyalgia may be precipitated by infections (Rea et al., 1999). Although tender points are a common, transient finding associated with acute infectious mononucleosis, fibromyalgia is an unusual long-term outcome (Rea et al., 1999). Hormonal changes may also affect tender points. For instance, Hapidou and Rollman (1998) documented that the number of tender points identified by palpation was greater in the follicular (postmenstrual) phase of the cycle as compared to the luteal (intermenstrual) phase in normally cycling women but not in users of oral contraceptives.

**thyroid microsomal antibodies:** In a cross-sectional study of forty-to forty-two-year-old men and women (737 and 771, respectively), Aarflot and Bruusgaard (1996) found that the prevalence of thyroid microsomal antibodies was significantly higher in persons with chronic widespread musculoskeletal complaints compared to those without (16.0 percent versus 7.3 percent). The increase was restricted to women, while thyroid function tests did not differ significantly between the two groups. Aarflot and Bruusgaard (1996) concluded that the association between chronic widespread musculoskeletal pain complaints and thyroid antibodies in women may reflect a subgroup of patients in which thyroid autoimmunity, rather than thyroid function, is important.

**tramadol:** In a double-blind crossover study of twelve fibromyalgia patients, Biasi et al. (1998) documented that during the first treatment cycle effective control of spontaneous pain was achieved with the centrally acting analgesic tramadol (100 mg ampule in 100 mL given intravenously in 15 minute doses), which determined a reduction of 20.6 percent while with the placebo spontaneous pain increased by 19.8 percent. As a cautionary note, Freye and Levy (2000) reported on a fibromyalgia patient who had taken tramadol for over one year and stopped abruptly, resulting in the development of classical abstinence-like symptoms within one week. Patients should be advised of such effects whenever they decide to stop intake or when their physician is planning to switch them to another medication. To avoid abstinence-like symptoms, doses should be slowly tapered down.

**trauma:** The concept that fibromyalgia may follow trauma is currently an area of intense debate within the medical field (Bohr, 1995; Ferrari and Kwan, 1999; Ferrari and Russell, 1998; Fishbain and Rosomoff, 1998; Link et al., 1996; "Nonarticular Rheumatism, Sports-Related Injuries, and Related Conditions," 1997; Pinals, 1997; Smith, 1998; White, Carette, et al., 2000; White, Ostbye, et al., 2000; Wigley, 1998), and Aaron et al. (1997) and Gardner (2000) stress that it is driven to a large extent by social and legal issues. Jenzer (1995) reported that whiplash injury to the cervical spine rarely results in disability, and, if so, it is only minor. Other authors support the lack of an association between whiplash injury and fibromyalgia (Cohen and Quintner, 1998; Gordon, 1997) despite an original article by Buskila et al. (1997).

In a study by White et al. (2000), random samples of 287 Canadian general practitioners, 160 orthopedists, 160 physiatrists, and 160 rheumatologists were surveyed as to whether they agreed with a diagnosis of fibromyalgia in a case scenario mailed to them, and what factors they considered to be important in the development of chronic, generalized posttraumatic pain. More recent medical school graduates were more likely to agree with the fibromyalgia diagnosis. Orthopedists (28.8 percent) were least likely to agree, while rheumatologists (83.0 percent) were most likely to agree. On multivariate analysis, three factors predicted agreement with the diagnosis of fibromyalgia: (1) number of fibromyalgia cases diagnosed by the respondent per week; (2) patient's sex; and (3) severity of initial injuries. Two factors predicted disagreement: (1) force of initial impact; and (2) patient's precollision psychiatric history. The authors concluded that future studies of the association between trauma and fibromyalgia should identify potential cases outside of specialty clinics, and baseline assessments should include some measurement of personality, stress, and precollision physical and mental health.

**treatment:** Treatment of fibromyalgia is largely empirical, palliative rather than curative, and symptom focused, although experience and small clinical studies have proved the efficacy of some pharmacological and nonpharmacological interventions from both conventional and alternative medicine sources, usually in a combination that is also sensitive to psychosocial factors (Akama, 2000; Bennett, 1995, 1996; Bennett et al., 1996; Burckhardt et al., 1998; Buskila, 1999; Clauw, 2000; Cohn, 2000; Eisinger and Dupond, 1996; Huppert, 2000; Keel, 1999; Keel et al., 1998; Lamberg, 1999; Langer, 1995; Leventhal, 1999; Littlejohn, 1995; Lloyd, 2000; Louis et al., 1998; Mason et al., 1998; McCain, 1996; Millea and Holloway, 2000; Muilenburg, 2000; Muller et al., 2000; Parziale, 1999; Reilly, 1999; Richards and Cleare, 2000; Rossy et al., 1999; Russell, 1996; Sandstrom and Keefe, 1998; Schachna and Littlejohn, 1999; Sim and Adams, 1999; Strobel et al., 1998; Tanum and Malt, 1995; Thomas et al., 1999; Turk et al., 1998; Wolfe, 2000; Zborovskii and Babaeva, 1996) (each therapeutic modality is discussed under the pertinent subheading). The presence of fibromyalgia affects the effectiveness of pharmacologic treatment of other diseases, such as rheumatoid arthritis (Wolfe, 1995). Development of treatment outcome assessment instruments is also an intense area of study (Alarcon and Bradley, 1998; Bakker et al., 1995; Finckh et al., 1998; Hewett et al., 1995; Rutten-van Molken et al., 1995; Zucker et al., 1997). Potential sources of bias in clinical trials include flaws in subject selection and group allocation, inadequate randomization, incomplete blinding, errors in outcome measurement, and inappropriate analysis of data (White and Harth, 1996).

**trigger points:** Trigger points are defined as areas of muscle that are painful to palpation and are characterized by the presence of taut bands and the generation of a referral pattern of pain, while tender points are areas of tenderness occurring in muscles, muscle-tendon junctions, bursa, or fat pads. Trigger points, which typically occur in a more restricted regional pattern than tender points, are indicative of myofascial pain syndrome (Borg-Stein and Stein, 1996; Schneider, 1995). In some patients the two phenomena may coexist, and overlapping syndromes can occur (Hong and Hsueh, 1996). In appropriately selected patients, it appears that myofascial trigger point injections can be helpful in decreasing pain and improving range of motion in conjunction with a comprehensive exercise and rehabilitation program (Hong and Hsueh, 1996; Jayson, 1996; Potter, 1997). In contrast to tender points, trigger points often respond to manual treatment methods, such as ischemic compression and various specific stretching techniques (Schneider, 1995).

**tryptophan:** Tryptophan is the amino acid precursor of serotonin, and the serotonergic system has been proposed to be connected to pathophysiology of fibromyalgia (*see* NEUROENDOCRINOLOGY). In agreement with the latter proposal, Schwarz et al. (1999) reported a strong negative correlation between serum levels of serotonin and tryptophan, and high serum concentrations of tryptophan showed a significant relation to low pain scores. Therapeutic administration of 5-hydroxytryptophan (5-HTP), the intermediate metabolite of the essential amino acid L-tryptophan in the biosynthesis of serotonin, has been shown to be effective in treating a wide variety of conditions, including depression, fibromyalgia, binge eating associated with obesity, chronic headaches, and insomnia (Birdsall, 1998).

**urine:** Fibromyalgia may be associated with an increase presence of bacteria in the urine (Xie et al., 1998), an observation that has not been studied broadly.

**venlafaxine:** Dwight et al. (1998) reported that out of eleven fibromyalgia patients who completed an open eight-week trial with the antidepressant venlafaxine, six (55 percent) experienced a greater or equal to 50 percent reduction of fibromyalgia symptoms. The presence of lifetime psychiatric disorders, particularly depressive and anxiety disorders, predicted a positive response to venlafaxine. These findings suggest that it is important to assess for comorbid psychiatric disorders in patients with fibromyalgia and that venlafaxine may be helpful to some of these patients (Dryson, 2000).

**virology:** Buchwald et al. (1996) reported that seroprevalence and/or geometric mean titer of antibodies to herpes simplex virus 1 and 2, rubella, adenovirus, human herpesvirus 6, Epstein-Barr virus, cytomegalovirus, and Coxsackie B virus, types 1-6 were not useful in evaluating patients presenting with chronic fatigue or in any subset of these patients, including those with chronic fatigue syndrome or fibromyalgia.

 **weather:** Quick (1997) points out that many people believe that weather conditions can influence joint pain, but science offers no proof. If the phenomenon were real, cause-and-effect mechanisms might provide clues that would aid joint pain treatment. Literature on the subject is sparse, conflicting, and vulnerable to bias, and further physiologic investigations are not likely to produce useful information. However, for patients who believe that weather can influence their pain, the causes may be unknown, but the effect is real (Quick, 1997).

 **zolpidem:** A dose-ranging, double-blind, placebo-controlled, modified crossover study by Moldofsky et al. (1996) concluded that although short-term treatment (sixteen nights) with zolpidem (5 to 15 mg orally at bedtime) does not affect the pain of fibromyalgia, it is useful for sleep and daytime energy in this patient population (Rothschild, 1997).

# Bibliography

*Abuse*

Alexander RW; Bradley LA; Alarcon GS; Triana-Alexander M; Aaron LA; Alberts KR; Martin MY; Stewart KE. (1998). Sexual and physical abuse in women with fibromyalgia: Association with outpatient health care utilization and pain medication usage. *Arthritis Care Research* 11(2):102-115.
Anderberg UM. (2000). [Fibromyalgia—probably a result of prolonged stress syndrome] Fibromyalgi—sannolikt ett resultat av langvarigt stressyndrom. *Lakartidningen* 97(21):2641-2642.
Anderberg UM; Marteinsdottir I; Theorell T; von Knorring L. (2000). The impact of life events in female patients with fibromyalgia and in female healthy controls. *European Psychiatry* 15(5):295-301.
Finestone HM; Stenn P; Davies F; Stalker C; Fry R; Koumanis J. (2000). Chronic pain and health care utilization in women with a history of childhood sexual abuse. *Child Abuse and Neglect* 24(4):547-556.
Goldberg RT; Pachas WN; Keith D. (1999). Relationship between traumatic events in childhood and chronic pain. *Disability and Rehabilitation* 21(1):23-30.
Walker EA; Keegan D; Gardner G; Sullivan M; Bernstein D; Katon WJ. (1997). Psychosocial factors in fibromyalgia compared with rheumatoid arthritis: II. Sexual, physical, and emotional abuse and neglect. *Psychosomatic Medicine* 59(6):572-577.
Winfield JB. (2000). Psychological determinants of fibromyalgia and related syndromes. *Current Reviews on Pain* 4(4):276-286.

*Acupuncture*

Acupuncture. (1997). *NIH Consensus Statement* 15(5):1-34.
Berman BM; Ezzo J; Hadhazy V; Swyers JP. (1999). Is acupuncture effective in the treatment of fibromyalgia? *Journal of Family Practice* 48(3):213-218.
Berman BM; Swyers JP. (1999). Complementary medicine treatments for fibromyalgia syndrome. *Baillieres Best Practice Research in Clinical Rheumatology* 13(3):487-492.
Berman BM; Swyers JP; Ezzo J. (2000). The evidence for acupuncture as a treatment for rheumatologic conditions. *Rheumatic Disease Clinics of North America* 26(1):103-115, ix-x.
Koenig C; Stevermer J. (1999). Acupuncture in the treatment of fibromyalgia. *Journal of Family Practice* 48(7):497.

Lee TL. (2000). Acupuncture and chronic pain management. *Annals of the Academy of Medicine of Singapore* 29(1):17-21.

Muller W; Pongratz D; Barlin E; Eich W; Farber L; Haus U; Lautenschlager J; Mense S; Neeck G; Offenbacher M; Spath M; Stratz T; Tolk J; Welzel D; Wiech K; Wohlgemuth M. (2000). The challenge of fibromyalgia: New approaches. *Scandinavian Journal of Rheumatology* (Suppl. 113):86.

NIH Consensus Conference. (1998). Acupuncture. *Journal of the American Medical Association* 280(17):1518-1524.

Offenbacher M; Stucki G. (2000). Physical therapy in the treatment of fibromyalgia. *Scandinavian Journal of Rheumatology* (Suppl. 113):78-85.

Ridgway K. (1999). Acupuncture as a treatment modality for back problems. *Veterinary Clinics of North America and Equine Practice* 15(1):211-221.

Sprott H; Franke S; Kluge H; Hein G. (1998). Pain treatment of fibromyalgia by acupuncture. *Rheumatology International* 18(1):35-36.

White A. (1995). The fibromyalgia syndrome. Electroacupuncture is a potentially valuable treatment. *British Medical Journal* 310(6991):1406.

*Affective Distress and Anxiety*

Celiker R; Borman P; Oktem F; Gokce-Kutsal Y; Basgoze O. (1997). Psychological disturbance in fibromyalgia: Relation to pain severity. *Clinical Rheumatology* 16(2):179-184.

Fischler B; Cluydts R; De Gucht Y; Kaufman L; De Meirleir K. (1997). Generalized anxiety disorder in chronic fatigue syndrome. *Acta Psychiatrica Scandinavica* 95(5):405-413.

Hallberg LR; Carlsson SG. (1998). Anxiety and coping in patients with chronic work-related muscular pain and patients with fibromyalgia. *European Journal of Pain* 2(4):309-319.

Kurtze N; Gundersen KT; Svebak S. (1998). The role of anxiety and depression in fatigue and patterns of pain among subgroups of fibromyalgia patients. *British Journal of Medical Psychology* 71(Pt. 2):185-194.

Kurtze N; Gundersen KT; Svebak S. (1999). Quality of life, functional disability and lifestyle among subgroups of fibromyalgia patients: The significance of anxiety and depression. *British Journal of Medical Psychology* 72(Pt. 4):471-484.

Walter B; Vaitl D; Frank R. (1998). Affective distress in fibromyalgia syndrome is associated with pain severity. *Zeitschrift Rheumatologie* 57 (Suppl. 2):101-104.

Wolfe F; Skevington SM. (2000). Measuring the epidemiology of distress: The rheumatology distress index. *Journal of Rheumatology* 27(8):2000-2009.

*Aging and Geriatrics*

Belilos E; Carsons S. (1998). Rheumatologic disorders in women. *Medicine Clinics of North America* 82(1):77-101.

Buckwalter JA; Lappin DR. (2000). The disproportionate impact of chronic arthralgia and arthritis among women. *Clinical Orthopedics* (372):159-168.
Goldenberg DL. (1996). Fibromyalgia, chronic fatigue syndrome, and myofascial pain. *Current Opinions in Rheumatology* 8(2):113-123.
Gowin KM. (2000). Diffuse pain syndromes in the elderly. *Rheumatic Disease Clinics of North America* 26(3):673-682.
Holland NW; Gonzalez EB. (1998). Soft tissue problems in older adults. *Clinical Geriatric Medicine* 14(3):601-611.
Meisler JG. (1999). Chronic pain conditions in women. *Journal of Women's Health* 8(3):313-320.
Michet CJ Jr; Evans JM; Fleming KC; O'Duffy JD; Jurisson ML; Hunder GG. (1995). Common rheumatologic diseases in elderly patients. *Mayo Clinic Proceedings* 70(12):1205-1214.

*Alcohol*

Eisinger J. (1998). Alcohol, thiamin and fibromyalgia. *Journal of the American College of Nutrition* 17(3):300-302.

*Allergy*

Tuncer T; Butun B; Arman M; Akyokus A; Doseyen A. (1997). Primary fibromyalgia and allergy. *Clinical Rheumatology* 16(1):9-12.

*Aloe*

Dykman KD; Tone C; Ford C; Dykman RA. (1998). The effects of nutritional supplements on the symptoms of fibromyalgia and chronic fatigue syndrome. *Integrative Physiological and Behavioral Science* 33(1):61-71.
Hadley SK; Petry JJ. (1999). Medicinal herbs: A primer for primary care. *Hospital Practice* 34(6):105-123.

*Alternative and Complementary Medicine*

Berman BM; Swyers JP. (1997). Establishing a research agenda for investigating alternative medical interventions for chronic pain. *Primary Care* 24(4):743-758.
Berman BM; Swyers JP. (1999). Complementary medicine treatments for fibromyalgia syndrome. *Baillieres Best Practice Research in Clinical Rheumatology* 13(3):487-492.
Dimmock S; Troughton PR; Bird HA. (1996). Factors predisposing to the resort of complementary therapies in patients with fibromyalgia. *Clinical Rheumatology* 15(5):478-482.
Fitzcharles MA; Esdaile JM. (1997). Nonphysician practitioner treatments and fibromyalgia syndrome. *Journal of Rheumatology* 24(5):937-940.

Hawkins D. (1998). Take two magnets and call me later. *US News and World Report* 125(22):86.

Nicassio PM; Schuman C; Kim J; Cordova A; Weisman MH. (1997). Psychosocial factors associated with complementary treatment use in fibromyalgia. *Journal of Rheumatology* 24(10):2008-2013.

Pioro-Boisset M; Esdaile JM; Fitzcharles MA. (1996). Alternative medicine use in fibromyalgia syndrome. *Arthritis Care Research* 9(1):13-17.

Rao JK; Mihaliak K; Kroenke K; Bradley J; Tierney WM; Weinberger M. (1999). Use of complementary therapies for arthritis among patients of rheumatologists. *Annals of Internal Medicine* 131(6):409-416.

### Amitriptyline

Bryson HM; Wilde MI. (1996). Amitriptyline. A review of its pharmacological properties and therapeutic use in chronic pain states. *Drugs and Aging* 8(6):459-476.

Carette S; Oakson G; Guimont C; Steriade M. (1995). Sleep electroencephalography and the clinical response to amitriptyline in patients with fibromyalgia. *Arthritis and Rheumatism* 38(9):1211-1217.

Godfrey RG. (1996). A guide to the understanding and use of tricyclic antidepressants in the overall management of fibromyalgia and other chronic pain syndromes. *Archives of Internal Medicine* 156(10):1047-1052.

Hannonen P; Malminiemi K; Yli-Kerttula U; Isomeri R; Roponen P. (1998). A randomized, double-blind, placebo-controlled study of moclobemide and amitriptyline in the treatment of fibromyalgia in females without psychiatric disorder. *British Journal of Rheumatology* 37(12):1279-1286.

Johnson SP. (1997). Fluoxetine and amitriptyline in the treatment of fibromyalgia. *Journal of Family Practice* 44(2):128-130.

Lautenschlager J. (2000). Present state of medication therapy in fibromyalgia syndrome. *Scandinavian Journal of Rheumatology* (Suppl. 113):32-36.

### Anticardiolipin Antibody

Gedalia A; Molina JF; Garcia CO; Doggett S; Espinoza LR; Gharavi AE. (1998). Anticardiolipin antibodies in childhood rheumatic disorders. *Lupus* 7(8):551-553.

### Antidepressants

Arnold LM; Keck PE Jr; Welge JA. (2000). Antidepressant treatment of fibromyalgia. A meta-analysis and review. *Psychosomatics* 41(2):104-113.

Baraczka K; Janko Z; Vargha K; Markus H. (1997). [Clinical experiences with the analgesic effects of citalopram] Klinikai tapasztalatok a citalopram fajdalomcsillapito hatasarol. *Orv Hetil* 138(41):2605-2607.

Fishbain D. (2000). Evidence-based data on pain relief with antidepressants. *Annals of Medicine* 32(5):305-316.

Godfrey RG. (1996). A guide to the understanding and use of tricyclic antidepressants in the overall management of fibromyalgia and other chronic pain syndromes. *Archives of Internal Medicine* 156(10):1047-1052.

Hannonen P; Malminiemi K; Yli-Kerttula U; Isomeri R; Roponen P. (1998). A randomized, double-blind, placebo-controlled study of moclobemide and amitriptyline in the treatment of fibromyalgia in females without psychiatric disorder. *British Journal of Rheumatology* 37(12):1279-1286.

Johnson SP. (1997). Fluoxetine and amitriptyline in the treatment of fibromyalgia. *Journal of Family Practice* 44(2):128-130.

Lautenschlager J. (2000). Present state of medication therapy in fibromyalgia syndrome. *Scandinavian Journal of Rheumatology* (Suppl. 113):32-36.

Maes M; Libbrecht I; Delmeire L; Lin A; De Clerck L; Scharpe S; Janca A. (1999). Changes in platelet alpha-2-adrenoceptors in fibromyalgia: Effects of treatment with antidepressants. *Neuropsychobiology* 40(3):129-133.

O'Malley PG; Balden E; Tomkins G; Santoro J; Kroenke K; Jackson JL. (2000). Treatment of fibromyalgia with antidepressants: A meta-analysis. *Journal of General Internal Medicine* 15(9):659-666.

O'Malley PG; Jackson JL; Santoro J; Tomkins G; Balden E; Kroenke K. (1999). Antidepressant therapy for unexplained symptoms and symptom syndromes. *Journal of Family Practice* 48(12):980-990.

Touchon J. (1995). [Use of antidepressants in sleep disorders: Practical considerations] Utilisation des antidepresseurs dans les troubles du sommeil: Considerations pratiques. *Encephale* 21 (Spec. No. 7):41-747.

*Antiganglioside Antibodies*

Klein R; Berg PA. (1995). High incidence of antibodies to 5-hydroxytryptamine, gangliosides and phospholipids in patients with chronic fatigue and fibromyalgia syndrome and their relatives: Evidence for a clinical entity of both disorders. *European Journal of Medical Research* 1(1):21-26.

*Antinuclear Antibodies*

Illei GG; Klippel JH. (1999). Why is the ANA result positive? *Bulletin of Rheumatic Diseases* 48(1):1-4.

Suarez-Almazor ME; Gonzalez-Lopez L; Gamez-Nava JI; Belseck E; Kendall CJ; Davis P. (1998). Utilization and predictive value of laboratory tests in patients referred to rheumatologists by primary care physicians. *Journal of Rheumatology* 25(10):1980-1985.

Tan EM; Feltkamp TE; Smolen JS; Butcher B; Dawkins R; Fritzler MJ; Gordon T; Hardin JA; Kalden JR; Lahita RG; Maini RN; McDougal JS; Rothfield NF; Smeenk RJ; Takasaki Y; Wiik A; Wilson MR; Koziol JA. (1997). Range of antinuclear antibodies in "healthy" individuals. *Arthritis and Rheumatism* 40(9):1601-1611.

*Antiphospholipid Antibodies*

Berg D; Berg LH; Couvaras J; Harrison H. (1999). Chronic fatigue syndrome and/or fibromyalgia as a variation of antiphospholipid antibody syndrome: An explanatory model and approach to laboratory diagnosis. *Blood Coagulation and Fibrinolysis* 10(7):435-438.

Gedalia A; Molina JF; Garcia CO; Doggett S; Espinoza LR; Gharavi AE. (1998). Anticardiolipin antibodies in childhood rheumatic disorders. *Lupus* 7(8):551-553.

Heller U; Becker EW; Zenner HP; Berg PA. (1998). [Incidence and clinical relevance of antibodies to phospholipids, serotonin and ganglioside in patients with sudden deafness and progressive inner ear hearing loss] Haufigkeit und klinische relevanz von antikorpern gegen phospholipide, serotonin und ganglioside bei patienten mit horsturz und progredienter innenohrschwerhorigkeit. *HNO* 46(6): 583-586.

Klein R; Berg PA. (1995). High incidence of antibodies to 5-hydroxytryptamine, gangliosides and phospholipids in patients with chronic fatigue and fibromyalgia syndrome and their relatives: Evidence for a clinical entity of both disorders. *European Journal of Medical Research* 1(1):21-26.

*Antipolymer Antibodies*

Angell M. (1997). Antipolymer antibodies, silicone breast implants, and fibromyalgia. *Lancet* 349(9059):1171-1172; discussion 1172-1173.

Edlavitch SA. (1997). Antipolymer antibodies, silicone breast implants, and fibromyalgia. *Lancet* 349(9059):1170.

Ellis TM; Hardt NS; Atkinson MA. (1997). Antipolymer antibodies, silicone breast implants, and fibromyalgia. *Lancet* 349(9059):1173.

Everson MP; Blackburn WD Jr. (1997). Antipolymer antibodies, silicone breast implants, and fibromyalgia. *Lancet* 349(9059):1171; discussion 1172-1173.

Korn JH. (1997). Antipolymer antibodies, silicone breast implants, and fibromyalgia. *Lancet* 349(9059):1171.

Lamm SH. (1997). Antipolymer antibodies, silicone breast implants, and fibromyalgia. *Lancet* 349(9059):1170-1171; discussion 1172-1173.

Wilson RB; Gluck OS; Tesser JR; Rice JC; Meyer A; Bridges AJ. (1999). Antipolymer antibody reactivity in a subset of patients with fibromyalgia correlates with severity. *Journal of Rheumatology* 26(2):402-407.

*Antiserotonin Antibodies*

Coplan JD; Tamir H; Calaprice D; DeJesus M; de la Nuez M; Pine D; Papp LA; Klein DF; Gorman JM. (1999). Plasma anti-serotonin and serotonin anti-idiotypic antibodies are elevated in panic disorder. *Neuropsychopharmacology* 20(4):386-391.

Heller U; Becker EW; Zenner HP; Berg PA. (1998). [Incidence and clinical relevance of antibodies to phospholipids, serotonin and ganglioside in patients with sudden deafness and progressive inner ear hearing loss] Haufigkeit und klinische relevanz von antikorpern gegen phospholipide, serotonin und ganglioside bei patienten mit horsturz und progredienter innenohrschwerhorigkeit. *HNO* 46(6): 583-586.

Klein R; Berg PA. (1995). High incidence of antibodies to 5-hydroxytryptamine, gangliosides and phospholipids in patients with chronic fatigue and fibromyalgia syndrome and their relatives: Evidence for a clinical entity of both disorders. *European Journal of Medical Research* 1(1):21-26.

Neeck G; Berg PA; Klein R. (1996). [Serotonin antibodies in fibromyalgia syndrome—expression of a neuroendocrinologic autoimmune disease?] Serotonin-antikorper beim fibromyalgie-syndrom—ausdruck einer neuroendokrinologischen autoimmunerkrankung? *Zeitschrift Rheumatologie (Journal of Rheumatology)* 55(1):63-65; 63,66; discussion 66-68.

Olin R; Klein R; Berg PA. (1998). A randomised double-blind 16-week study of ritanserin in fibromyalgia syndrome: Clinical outcome and analysis of autoantibodies to serotonin, gangliosides and phospholipids. *Clinical Rheumatology* 17(2):89-94.

## Artists and Musicians

Hingtgen CM. (1999). The painful perils of a pair of pianists: The chronic pain of Clara Schumann and Sergei Rachmaninov. *Seminars in Neurology* 19 (Suppl. 1): 29-34.

Martinez-Lavin M; Amigo MC; Coindreau J; Canoso J. (2000). Fibromyalgia in Frida Kahlo's life and art. *Arthritis and Rheumatism* 43(3):708-709.

Potter PJ; Jones IC. (1995). Medical problems affecting musicians. *Canadian Family Physician* 41:2121-2128.

## Ascorbigen

Bramwell B; Ferguson S; Scarlett N; Macintosh A. (2000). The use of ascorbigen in the treatment of fibromyalgia patients: A preliminary trial. *Alternative Medical Reviews* 5(5):455-462.

## Attributions

Neerinckx E; Van Houdenhove B; Lysens R; Vertommen H; Onghena P. (2000). Attributions in chronic fatigue syndrome and fibromyalgia syndrome in tertiary care. *Journal of Rheumatology* 27(4):1051-1055.

## Autoimmune Fatigue Syndrome

Itoh Y; Fukunaga Y; Igarashi T; Imai T; Yoshida J; Tsuchiya M; Fujino O; Murakami M; Yamamoto M. (1998). Autoimmunity in chronic fatigue syndrome in children. *Japanese Journal of Rheumatology* 8(4):427-429.

Itoh Y; Hamada H; Imai T; Saki T; Igarashi T; Yuge K; Fukunaga Y; Yamamoto M; (1997). Antinuclear antibodies in children with chronic nonspecific complaints. *Autoimmunity* 25(4):243-250.

Itoh Y; Igarashi T; Tatsuma N; Imai T; Yoshida J; Tsuchiya M; Murakami M; Fukunaga Y. (1999). [Autoimmune fatigue syndrome and fibromyalgia syndrome]. *Nippon Ika Daigaku Zasshi* 66(4):239-244.

Itoh Y; Igarashi T; Tatsuma N; Imai T; Yoshida J; Tsuchiya M; Murakami M; Fukunaga Y. (2000). Immunogenetic background of patients with autoimmune fatigue syndrome. *Autoimmunity* 32:193-197.

## Autonomic Dysfunction

Bou-Holaigah I; Calkins H; Flynn JA; Tunin C; Chang HC; Kan JS; Rowe PC. (1997). Provocation of hypotension and pain during upright tilt table testing in adults with fibromyalgia. *Clinical and Experimental Rheumatology* 15(3):239-246.

Cohen H; Neumann L; Shore M; Amir M; Cassuto Y; Buskila D. (2000). Autonomic dysfunction in patients with fibromyalgia: Application of power spectral analysis of heart rate variability. *Seminars in Arthritis and Rheumatism* 29(4):217-227.

Kelemen J; Lang E; Balint G; Trocsanyi M; Muller W. (1998). Orthostatic sympathetic derangement of baroreflex in patients with fibromyalgia. *Journal of Rheumatology* 25(4):823-825.

Martinez-Lavin M; Hermosillo AG. (2000). Autonomic nervous system dysfunction may explain the multisystem features of fibromyalgia. *Seminars in Arthritis and Rheumatism* 29(4):197-199.

Martinez-Lavin M; Hermosillo AG; Mendoza C; Ortiz R; Cajigas JC; Pineda C; Nava A; Vallejo M. (1997). Orthostatic sympathetic derangement in subjects with fibromyalgia. *Journal of Rheumatology* 24(4):714-718.

Martinez-Lavin M; Hermosillo AG; Rosas M; Soto ME. (1998). Circadian studies of autonomic nervous balance in patients with fibromyalgia: A heart rate variability analysis. *Arthritis and Rheumatism* 41(11):1966-1971.

Sendrowski DP; Buker EA; Gee SS. (1997). An investigation of sympathetic hypersensitivity in chronic fatigue syndrome. *Optometry and Visual Sciences* 74(8):660-663.

Tougas G. (1999). The autonomic nervous system in functional bowel disorders. *Canadian Journal of Gastroenterology* 13 (Suppl. A):15A-17A.

Wilke WS; Fouad-Tarazi FM; Cash JM; Calabrese LH. (1998). The connection between chronic fatigue syndrome and neurally mediated hypotension. *Cleveland Clinic Journal of Medicine* 65(5):261-266.

### Behcet's Syndrome

Yavuz S; Fresko I; Hamuryudan V; Yurdakul S; Yazici H. (1998). Fibromyalgia in Behcet's syndrome. *Journal of Rheumatology* 25(11):2219-2220.

### Benzodiazepine-Induced Hip Fracture

Robb-Nicholson C. (1998). I read in your June 1997 publication that one of the risk factors for hip fracture is current use of long-acting benzodiazepines. Could you list exactly which medications these are? I take Xanax and doxepin for fibromyalgia. My pharmacist could find no evidence that either of these drugs depletes bone calcium. How do they place me at increased risk for osteoporosis? *Harvard Women's Health Watch* 5(5):8.

### Biofeedback

Buckelew SP; Conway R; Parker J; Deuser WE; Read J; Witty TE; Hewett JE; Minor M; Johnson JC; Van Male L; McIntosh MJ; Nigh M; Kay DR. (1998). Biofeedback/relaxation training and exercise interventions for fibromyalgia: A prospective trial. *Arthritis Care Research* 11(3):196-209.

Mur E; Drexler A; Gruber J; Hartig F; Gunther V. (1999). [Electromyography biofeedback therapy in fibromyalgia] EMG-biofeedback-therapie bei fibromyalgie. *Wien Medizinishe Wochenschrift* 149(19-20):561-563.

Sarnoch H; Adler F; Scholz OB. (1997). Relevance of muscular sensitivity, muscular activity, and cognitive variables for pain reduction associated with EMG biofeedback in fibromyalgia. *Perception and Motor Skills* 84(3 Pt. 1):1043-1050.

### Borna Disease Virus

Kitani T; Kuratsune H; Fuke I; Nakamura Y; Nakaya T; Asahi S; Tobiume M; Yamaguti M; Machii T; Inagi R; Yamanishi K; Ikuta K. (1996). Possible correlation between borna disease virus infection and Japanese patients with chronic fatigue syndrome. *Microbiology and Immunology* 40(6):459-462.

Nakaya T; Kuratsune H; Kitani T; Ikuta K. (1997). Demonstration on borna disease virus in patients with chronic fatigue syndrome. *Nippon Rinsho—Japanese Journal of Clinical Medicine* 55(11):3064-3071.

Nakaya T; Takahashi H; Nakamura Y; Asahi S; Tobiume M; Kuratsune H; Kitani T; Yamanishi K; Ikuta K. (1996). Demonstration of Borna disease virus RNA in peripheral blood mononuclear cells derived from Japanese patients with chronic fatigue syndrome. *FEBS Letters* 378(2):145-149.

Wittrup IH; Christensen LS; Jensen B; Danneskiold-Samsoe B; Bliddal H; Wiik (2000). A. Search for Borna disease virus in Danish fibromyalgia patients. *Scandinavian Journal of Rheumatology* 29:387-390.

### Botulinum Toxin

Paulson GW; Gill W. (1996). Botulinum toxin is unsatisfactory therapy for fibromyalgia. *Movement Disorders* 11(4):459.

### Breast Implants

Angell M. (1997). Antipolymer antibodies, silicone breast implants, and fibromyalgia. *Lancet* 349(9059):1171-1172; discussion 1172-1173.

Blackburn WD Jr; Grotting JC; Everson MP. (1997). Lack of evidence of systemic inflammatory rheumatic disorders in symptomatic women with breast implants. *Plastic and Reconstructive Surgery* 99(4):1054-1060.

Bridges AJ; Anderson JD; Burns DE; Kemple K; Kaplan JD; Lorden T. (1996). Autoantibodies in patients with silicone implants. *Current Topics in Microbiology and Immunology* 210:317-322.

Brown SL; Langone JJ; Brinton LA. (1998). Silicone breast implants and autoimmune disease. *Journal of the American Medical Women's Association* 53(1): 21-24, 40.

Cuellar ML; Gluck O; Molina JF; Gutierrez S; Garcia C; Espinoza R. (1995). Silicone breast implant—associated musculoskeletal manifestations. *Clinical Rheumatology* 14(6):667-672.

Edlavitch SA. (1997). Antipolymer antibodies, silicone breast implants, and fibromyalgia. *Lancet* 349(9059):1170.

Ellis TM; Hardt NS; Atkinson MA. (1997). Antipolymer antibodies, silicone breast implants, and fibromyalgia. *Lancet* 349(9059):1173.

Everson MP; Blackburn WD Jr. (1997). Antipolymer antibodies, silicone breast implants, and fibromyalgia. *Lancet* 349(9059):1171; discussion 1172-1173.

Friis S; Mellemkjaer L; McLaughlin JK; Breiting V; Kjaer SK; Blot W; Olsen JH. (1997). Connective tissue disease and other rheumatic conditions following breast implants in Denmark. *Annals of Plastic Surgery* 39(1):1-8.

Fuchs H; Johnson JS; Sergent JS. (1995). Still more on breast implants and connective-tissue diseases. *New England Journal of Medicine* 333(8):526.

Korn JH. (1997). Antipolymer antibodies, silicone breast implants, and fibromyalgia. *Lancet* 349(9059):1171.

Lai S; Goldman JA; Child AH; Engel A; Lamm SH. (2000). Fibromyalgia, hypermobility, and breast implants. *Journal of Rheumatology* 27(9):2237-2241.

Lamm SH. (1997). Antipolymer antibodies, silicone breast implants, and fibromyalgia. *Lancet* 349(9059):1170-1171; discussion 1172-1173.

Levenson T; Greenberger PA; Murphy R. (1996). Peripheral blood eosinophilia, hyperimmunoglobulinemia A and fatigue: Possible complications following rupture of silicone breast implants. *Annals of Allergy, Asthma, and Immunology* 77(2):119-122.

Levine P; Clauw DJ; Claman HC; Robertson AD; Ketch L. (2000). Silicone breast implants, chronic fatigue syndrome and fibromyalgia. *Journal of Chronic Fatigue Syndrome* 7(1):53-74.

Martin L. (1999). Silicone breast implants: The saga continues. *Journal of Rheumatology* 26(5):1020-1021.

Nyren O; Yin L; Josefsson S; McLaughlin JK; Blot WJ; Engqvist M; Hakelius L; Boice JD Jr; Adami HO. (1998). Risk of connective tissue disease and related disorders among women with breast implants: A nation-wide retrospective cohort study in Sweden. *British Medical Journal* 316(7129):417-422.

Peters W; Smith D; Fornasier V; Lugowski S; Ibanez D. (1997). An outcome analysis of 100 women after explantation of silicone gel breast implants. *Annals of Plastic Surgery* 39(1):9-19.

Romano TJ. (1996). Breast implants and connective-tissue disease. *Journal of the American Medical Association* 276(2):102; discussion 103.

Rosenberg NL. (1996). The neuromythology of silicone breast implants. *Neurology* 46(2):308-314.

Silverman S; Gluck O; Silver D; Tesser J; Wallace D; Neumann K; Metzger A; Morris R. (1996). The prevalence of autoantibodies in symptomatic and asymptomatic patients with breast implants and patients with fibromyalgia. *Current Topics in Microbiology and Immunology* 210:277-282.

Thomas WO III; Harper LL; Wong SW; Michalski JP; Harris CN; Moore JT; Rodning CB. (1997). Explanation of silicone breast implants. *American Surgery* 63(5):421-429.

Vasey FB. (1997). Clinical experience with systemic illness in women with silicone breast implants: Comment on the editorial by Rose. *Arthritis and Rheumatism* 40(8):1545.

Vasey FB; Aziz N. (1995). Breast implants and connective-tissue diseases. *New England Journal of Medicine* 333(21):1423; discussion 1424.

Wolfe F. (1999). "Silicone-related symptoms" are common in patients with fibromyalgia: No evidence for a new disease. *Journal of Rheumatology* 26(5):1172-1175.

Wolfe F; Anderson J. (1999). Silicone-filled breast implants and the risk of fibromyalgia and rheumatoid arthritis. *Journal of Rheumatology* 26(9):2025-2028.

Young VL; Nemecek JR; Schwartz BD; Phelan DL; Schorr MW. (1995). HLA typing in women with breast implants. *Plastic and Reconstructive Surgery* 96(7): 1497-1519; discussion 1520.

## Breathing

Alvarez-Lario B; Viejo Banuelos JL. (1997). [Sleep respiratory disorders in fibromyalgia syndrome] Trastornos respiratorios del sueno en el sindrome de fibromialgia. *Archives of Bronconeumology* 33(3):143-147.
Ozgocmen S; Ardicoglu O. (1999). Reduced chest expansion in primary fibromyalgia syndrome. *Yonsei Medical Journal* 40(1):90-91.
Sergi M; Rizzi M; Braghiroli A; Puttini PS; Greco M; Cazzola M; Andreoli A. (1999). Periodic breathing during sleep in patients affected by fibromyalgia syndrome. *European Respiratory Journal* 14(1):203-208.
Weiss DJ; Kreck T; Albert RK. (1998). Dyspnea resulting from fibromyalgia. *Chest* 113(1):246-249.

## Calcitonin

Bessette L; Carette S; Fossel AH; Lew RA. (1998). A placebo controlled crossover trial of subcutaneous salmon calcitonin in the treatment of patients with fibromyalgia. *Scandinavian Journal of Rheumatology* 27(2):112-116.

## Cancer Chemotherapy

Simonson N. (1996). [Can tamoxifen relieve fibromyalgia?] Kan tamoxifen lindra fibromyalgi? *Lakartidningen* 93(5):340.
Warner E; Keshavjee al-N; Shupak R; Bellini A. (1997). Rheumatic symptoms following adjuvant therapy for breast cancer. *American Journal of Clinical Oncology* 20(3):322-326.

## Carpal Tunnel Syndrome

Cimmino MA; Parisi M; Moggiana G; Accardo S. (1996). The association between fibromyalgia and carpal tunnel syndrome in the general population. *Annals of Rheumatic Diseases* 55(10):780.
Perez-Ruiz F; Calabozo M; Alonso-Ruiz A; Ruiz-Lucea E. (1997). Fibromyalgia and carpal tunnel syndrome. *Annals of Rheumatic Diseases* 56(7):438-439.
Straub TA. (1999). Endoscopic carpal tunnel release: A prospective analysis of factors associated with unsatisfactory results. *Arthroscopy* 15(3):269-274.

## Chemical Intolerance

Bell IR; Baldwin CM; Russek LG; Schwartz GE; Hardin EE. (1998). Early life stress, negative paternal relationships, and chemical intolerance in middle-aged women: Support for a neural sensitization model. *Journal of Women's Health* 7(9):1135-1147.

Bell IR; Baldwin CM; Schwartz GE. (1998). Illness from low levels of environmental chemicals: Relevance to chronic fatigue syndrome and fibromyalgia. *American Journal of Medicine* 105(3A):74S-82S.

Bell IR; Patarca R; Baldwin CM; Klimas NG; Schwartz GE; Hardin EE. (1998). Serum neopterin and somatization in women with chemical intolerance, depressives, and normals. *Neuropsychobiology* 38(1):13-18.

Bell IR; Szarek MJ; Dicenso DR; Baldwin CM; Schwartz GE; Bootzin RR. (1999). Patterns of waking EEG spectral power in chemically intolerant individuals during repeated chemical exposures. *International Journal of Neurosciences* 97(1-2):41-59.

Csef H. (1998). [The non-specific environmental syndromes MCS (multiple chemical sensitivity), IEI (idiopathic environmental intolerance) and SBS (sick building syndrome)] Die unspezifischen umweltsyndrome MCS, IEI und SBS klinische bilder und therapieansatze. *Fortschrift Medizin* 116(33):18-20, 22, 24.

Fiedler N; Kipen HM; DeLuca J; Kelly-McNeil K; Natelson B. (1996). A controlled comparison of multiple chemical sensitivities and chronic fatigue syndrome. *Psychosomatic Medicine* 58(1):38-49.

Gibson PR; Cheavens J; Warren ML. (1998). Social support in persons with self-reported sensitivity to chemicals. *Research in Nursing and Health* 21(2):103-115.

Lohmann K; Prohl A; Schwarz E. (1996). Multiple chemical sensitivity disorder in patients with neurotoxic illnesses. *Gesundheitswesen* 58(6):322-331.

Miller CS. (1999). Are we on the threshold of a new theory of disease? Toxicant-induced loss of tolerance and its relationship to addiction and abdiction. *Toxicology and Industrial Health* 15(3-4):284-294.

Multiple chemical sensitivity: A 1999 consensus. (1999). *Archives of Environmental Health* 54(3):147-149.

Rowat SC. (1999). Paraoxonase/MCS. *Environmental Health Perspectives* 107(8):A395.

Shanklin DR; Stevens MV; Hall MF; Smalley DL. (2000). Environmental immunogens and T-cell-mediated responses in fibromyalgia: Evidence for immune dysregulation and determinants of granuloma formation. *Experimental Molecular Pathology* 69(2):102-118.

Slotkoff AT; Radulovic DA; Clauw DJ. (1997). The relationship between fibromyalgia and the multiple chemical sensitivity syndrome. *Scandinavian Journal of Rheumatology* 26(5):364-367.

Weiss B. (1998). Neurobehavioral properties of chemical sensitivity syndromes. *Neurotoxicology* 19(2):259-268.

Ziem G; McTamney J. (1997). Profile of patients with chemical injury and sensitivity. *Environmental Health Perspectives* 105 (Suppl. 2):417-436.

## Chiari Malformation

Bradley LA; Alarcon GS. (1999). Is Chiari malformation associated with increased levels of substance P and clinical symptoms in persons with fibromyalgia? *Arthritis and Rheumatism* 42(12):2731-2732.

Muller W; Kelemen J; Stratz T. (1998). Spinal factors in the generation of fibromyalgia syndrome. *Zeitschrift Rheumatologie* 57 (Suppl. 2):36-42.

## Chiropractic Treatment

Blunt KL; Rajwani MH; Guerriero RC. (1997). The effectiveness of chiropractic management of fibromyalgia patients: A pilot study. *Journal of Manipulative Physiological Therapy* 20(6):389-399.

Hains G; Hains F. (2000). A combined ischemic compression and spinal manipulation in the treatment of fibromyalgia: A preliminary estimate of dose and efficacy. *Journal of Manipulative Physiological Therapy* 23(4):225-230.

Harper A; Liu D. (1998). The effectiveness of chiropractic management of fibromyalgia patients: A pilot study. *Journal of Manipulative Physiological Therapy* 21(6):429.

Schneider M. (1998). The effectiveness of chiropractic management of fibromyalgia patients. *Journal of Manipulative Physiological Therapy* 21(4):307.

## Chlamydia

Machtey I. (1997). *Chlamydia pneumoniae* antibodies in myalgia of unknown cause (including fibromyalgia). *British Journal of Rheumatology* 36(10):1134.

## Chlorella Pyrenoidosa

Merchant RE; Carmack CA; Wise CM. (2000). Nutritional supplementation with *Chlorella pyrenoidosa* for patients with fibromyalgia syndrome: A pilot study. *Phytotherapy Research* 14(3):167-173.

## Chronic Fatigue Syndrome

Baschetti R. (1997). Etiology of chronic fatigue syndrome. *American Journal of Medicine* 102(4):422-423.

Bazelmans E; Vercoulen JH; Swanink CM; Fennis JF; Galama JM; van Weel C; van der Meer JW; Bleijenberg G. (1999). Chronic fatigue syndrome and primary fibromyalgia syndrome as recognized by GPs. *Family Practice* 16(6):602-604.

Bertolin JM; Calvo J. (1997). Chronic fatigue syndrome. To be or not to be? *Medicina Clinica* 108(15):577-579.

Buchwald D. (1996). Fibromyalgia and chronic fatigue syndrome: Similarities and differences. *Rheumatic Disease Clinics of North America* 22(2):219-243.

Buchwald D; Umali J; Pearlman T; Kith P; Ashley R; Wener M. (1996). Post-infectious chronic fatigue: A distinct syndrome? *Clinical Infectious Diseases* 23(2):385-387.

Butler C; Rollnick S. (1996). Missing the meaning and provoking resistance: A case of myalgic encephalomyelitis. *Family Practice* 13(1):106-109.

Caplan C. (1998). Chronic fatigue syndrome or just plain tired? *Canadian Medical Association Journal* 159(5):519-520.

Chalder T; Power MJ; Wessely S. (1996). Chronic fatigue in the community: A question of attribution. *Psychological Medicine* 26(4):791-800.

Chester AC. (1997). Chronic fatigue syndrome criteria in patients with other forms of unexplained chronic fatigue. *Journal of Psychiatric Research* 31(1):45-50.

Cheung F; Lin KM. (1997). Neurasthenia, depression and somatoform disorder in a Chinese-Vietnamese woman migrant. *Culture, Medicine and Psychiatry* 21(2):247-58.

Clauw DJ; Chrousos GP. (1997). Chronic pain and fatigue syndromes: Overlapping clinical and neuroendocrine features and potential pathogenic mechanisms. *Neuroimmunomodulation* 4(3):134-153.

Cook NF; Boore JR. (1997). Managing patients suffering from acute and chronic fatigue. *British Journal of Nursing* 6(14):811-815.

de Loos WS. (1997). Chronic fatigue syndrome: Fatigue of unknown origin. *European Journal of Clinical Investigation* 27(4):268-269.

Delbanco TL; Daley J; Hartman EE. (1998). A 56-year-old woman with chronic fatigue syndrome, 1 year later. *Journal of the American Medical Association* 280(4):372.

DeLuca J; Johnson SK; Ellis SP; Natelson BH. (1997). Sudden vs. gradual onset of chronic fatigue syndrome differentiates individuals on cognitive and psychiatric measures. *Journal of Psychiatric Research* 31(1):83-90.

Demitrack MA. (1998). Chronic fatigue syndrome and fibromyalgia. Dilemmas in diagnosis and clinical management. *Psychiatry Clinics of North America* 21(3):671-692, viii.

Dickinson CJ. (1997). Chronic fatigue syndrome: Aetiological aspects. *European Journal of Clinical Investigation* 27(4):257-267.

Dyck D; Allen S; Barron J; Marchi J; Price BA; Spavor L; Tateishi S. (1996). Management of chronic fatigue syndrome: Case study. *AAOHN Journal* 44(2):85-92.

Evengard B; Nilsson CG; Lindh G; Lindquist L; Eneroth P; Fredrikson S; Terenius L; Henriksson KG. (1998). Chronic fatigue syndrome differs from fibromyalgia. No evidence for elevated substance P levels in cerebrospinal fluid of patients with chronic fatigue syndrome. *Pain* 78(2):153-155.

Franklin A. (1998). How I manage chronic fatigue syndrome. *Archives of Disease in Childhood* 79(4):375-378.

Fuller NS; Morrison RE. (1998). Chronic fatigue syndrome: Helping patients cope with this enigmatic illness. *Postgraduate Medicine* 103(1):175-176, 179-184.

Gompels MM; Spickett GP. (1996). Chronic fatigue, arthralgia, and malaise. *Annals of Rheumatic Diseases* 55(8):502-503.

Goshorn RK. (1998). Chronic fatigue syndrome: A review for clinicians. *Seminars in Neurology* 18(2):237-242.

Hadler NM. (1997). Fibromyalgia, chronic fatigue, and other iatrogenic diagnostic algorithms: Do some labels escalate illness in vulnerable patients? *Postgraduate Medicine* 102(2):161-162, 165-166, 171-172.

Hakimi R. (1996). Chronic fatigue syndrome—also an insurance medicine problem. *Versicherungsmedizin* 48(2):59-61.

Harrigan P. (1998). Controversy continues over chronic fatigue syndrome. *Lancet* 351(9102):574.

Hartz AJ; Kuhn EM; Levine PH. (1998). Characteristics of fatigued persons associated with features of chronic fatigue syndrome. *Journal of Chronic Fatigue Syndrome* 4(3):71-97.

Hausotter W. (1996). Expert assessment of chronic fatigue syndrome. *Versicherungsmedizin* 48(2):57-59.

Heyll U; Wachauf P; Senger V; Diewitz M. (1997). Definition of "chronic fatigue syndrome" (CFS). *Medizinische Klinik* 92(4):221-227.

Hickie I; Hadzi-Pavlovic D; Ricci C. (1997). Reviving the diagnosis of neurasthenia. *Psychological Medicine* 27(5):989-994.

Hickie I; Lloyd A; Wakefield D; Ricci C. (1996). Is there a postinfection fatigue syndrome? *Australian Family Physician* 25(12):1847-1852.

Hoffmann A; Linder R; Kroger B; Schnabel A; Kruger GR. (1996). [Fibromyalgia syndrome and chronic fatigue syndrome. Similarities and differences] Fibromyalgie-syndrom und chronic-fatigue-syndrom. gemeinsamkeiten und unterschiede. *Deutsche Medizin Wochenschrift* 121(38):1165-1168.

Houde SC; Kampfe-Leacher R. (1997). Chronic fatigue syndrome: An update for clinicians in primary care. *Nurse Practitioner* 22(7):30, 35-36, 39-40.

Joyce J; Rabe-Hesketh S; Wessely S. (1998). Reviewing the reviews: The example of chronic fatigue syndrome. *Journal of the American Medical Association* 280(3):264-266.

Kenner C. (1998). Fibromyalgia and chronic fatigue: The holistic perspective. *Holistic Nursing Practice* 12(3):55-63.

Komaroff AL. (1997). A 56-year-old woman with chronic fatigue syndrome. *Journal of the American Medical Association* 278(14):1179-1185.

Komaroff AL; Buchwald DS. (1998). Chronic fatigue syndrome: An update. *Annual Review of Medicine* 49:1-13.

Komaroff AL; Fagioli LR; Geiger AM; Doolittle TH; Lee J; Kornish RJ; Gleit MA; Guerriero RT. (1996). An examination of the working case definition of chronic fatigue syndrome. *American Journal of Medicine* 100(1):56-64.

Lapp CW; Hyman HL. (1997). Diagnosis of chronic fatigue syndrome. *Archives of Internal Medicine* 157(22):2663-2664.

Layzer RB: (1998). Asthenia and the chronic fatigue syndrome. *Muscle and Nerve* 21(12):1609-1611.

Lee P. (1998). Recent developments in chronic fatigue syndrome. *American Journal of Medicine* 105(3A):1S.

Levine PH. (1998a). Chronic fatigue syndrome comes of age. *American Journal of Medicine* 105(3A):2S-6S.

Levine PH. (1998b). What we know about chronic fatigue syndrome and its relevance to the practicing physician. *American Journal of Medicine* 105(3A):100S-103S.

Lieb K; Dammann G; Berger M; Bauer J. (1996). Chronic fatigue syndrome. Definition, diagnostic measures and therapeutic possibilities. *Nervenarzt* 67(9):711-720.

Lipkin DM; Papernik M; Kaan R. (1997). Chronic fatigue. *American Journal of Psychiatry* 154(9):1322.

Lloyd AR. (1998). Chronic fatigue and chronic fatigue syndrome: Shifting boundaries and attributions. *American Journal of Medicine* 105(3A):7S-10S.

MacDonald KL; Osterholm MT; LeDell KH; White KE; Schenck CH; Chao CC; Persing DH; Johnson RC; Barker JM; Peterson PK. (1996). A case-control study to assess possible triggers and cofactors in chronic fatigue syndrome. *American Journal of Medicine* 100(5):548-554.

Massey RU. (1996). Neurasthenia, psychasthenia, CFS, and related mattters. *Connecticut Medicine* 60(10):627-628.

McCluskey DR. (1998). Chronic fatigue syndrome: Its cause and a strategy for management. *Comprehensive Therapy* 24(8):357-363.

Mellergard M. (1997). Only extremely tired? *Ugeskrift for Laeger* 159(31):4769.

Miro O; Font C; Fernandez-Sola J; Casademont J; Pedrol E; Grau JM; Urbano-Marquez A. (1997). Chronic fatigue syndrome: Study of the clinical course of 28 cases. *Medicina Clinica* 108(15):561-565.

Mulube M. (1996). Myths dispelled about chronic fatigue syndrome. *British Medical Journal* 313(7061):839.

Nisenbaum R; Reyes M; Mawle AC; Reeves WC. (1998). Factor analysis of unexplained severe fatigue and interrelated symptoms: Overlap with criteria for chronic fatigue syndrome. *American Journal of Epidemiology* 148(1):72-77.

Patarca-Montero, R. (2000). *The Concise Encyclopedia of Chronic Fatigue Syndrome*. Binghamton, NY: The Haworth Press, Inc.

Plioplys AV; Plioplys S; Davis JS IV. (1997). Meeting the frustrations of chronic fatigue syndrome. *Hospital Practice* 32(6):147-150, 153-156, 160-161.

Ross E. (1996). The history and treatment of chronic fatigue syndrome. *Nursing Times* 92(44):34-36.

Salit IE. (1996). The chronic fatigue syndrome: A position paper. *Journal of Rheumatology* 23(3):540-544.

Salit IE. (1997). Precipitating factors for the chronic fatigue syndrome. *Journal of Psychiatric Research* 31(1):59-65.

Sharpe M; Chalder T; Palmer I; Wessely S. (1997). Chronic fatigue syndrome: A practical guide to assessment and management. *General Hospital Psychiatry* 19(3):185-199.

Sibbald B. (1998). Chronic fatigue syndrome comes out of the closet. *Canadian Medical Association Journal* 159(5):537-541.

Simpson M; Bennett A; Holland P. (1997). Chronic fatigue syndrome/myalgic encephalomyelitis as a twentieth-century disease: Analytic challenges. *Journal of Analytical Psychology* 42(2):191-199.

Streeten DH. (1998). The nature of chronic fatigue. *Journal of the American Medical Association* 280(12):1094-1095.

Suarez-Lozano I. (1997). Isolated general malaise of unknown origin: A new syndrome. *Anales de Medicina Interna* 14(4):209-210.

Teran Diaz E. (1996). *Anales de Medicina Interna* 13(10):467-470.

Tuck I; Human N. (1998). The experience of living with chronic fatigue syndrome. *Journal of Psychosocial Nursing and Mental Health Services* 36(2):15-19.

van der Meer JW; Elving LD. (1997). Chronic fatigue—cured with 23 I's. *Nederlands Tijdschrift voor Geneeskunde* 141(31):1505-1507.

van der Meer JW; Rijken PM; Bleijenberg G; Thomas S; Hinloopen RJ; Bensing JM. (1997). Indications for management in long-term, physically unexplained fatigue symptoms. *Nederlands Tijdschrift voor Geneeskunde* 141(31):1516-1519.

van Waveren EK. (1996). The rise and fall of the chronic fatigue syndrome as defined by Holmes et al. *Medical Hypotheses* 46(2):63-66.

Wessely S. (1996). Chronic fatigue syndrome. Summary of a report of a joint committee of the Royal College of Physicians, Psychiatrists and General Practitioners. *Journal of the Royal College of Physicians of London* 30(6):497-504.

Wessely S. (1997). Chronic fatigue syndrome: A 20th century illness? *Scandinavian Journal of Work, Environment and Health* 23 (Suppl. 3):17-34.

Wessely S. (1998). The epidemiology of chronic fatigue syndrome. *Epidemiologia e Psichiatria Sociale* 7(1):10-24.

White KP; Speechley M; Harth M; Ostbye T. (2000). Co-existence of chronic fatigue syndrome with fibromyalgia syndrome in the general population. A controlled study. *Scandinavian Journal of Rheumatology* 29(1):44-51.

Ziem G; Donnay A. (1995). Chronic fatigue, fibromyalgia, and chemical sensitivity: Overlapping disorders. *Archives of Internal Medicine* 155(17):1913.

## *Cogan I Syndrome*

Zierhut M; Schlote T; Stubiger N; Daikeler T; Kotter I; Bless D; Koitschev A. (2000). [Cogan I syndrome: Clinical aspects, therapy and prognosis] Cogan I-syndrom: klinik, therapie und prognose. *Ophthalmologe* 97(3):197-202.

*Cognitive-Behavioral Therapy*

Bradley LA; Alberts KR. (1999). Psychological and behavioral approaches to pain management for patients with rheumatic disease. *Rheumatic Diseases Clinics of North America* 25(1):215-232, viii.

Callahan LF; Blalock SJ. (1997). Behavioral and social research in rheumatology. *Current Opinion in Rheumatology* 9(2):126-132.

Goossens ME; Rutten-van Molken MP; Leidl RM; Bos SG; Vlaeyen JW; Teeken-Gruben NJ. (1996). Cognitive-educational treatment of fibromyalgia: A randomized clinical trial. II. Economic evaluation. *Journal of Rheumatology* 23(7):1246-1254.

Goossens ME; Rutten-van Molken MP; Vlaeyen JW; van der Linden SM. (2000). The cost diary: A method to measure direct and indirect costs in cost-effectiveness research. *Journal of Clinical Epidemiology* 53(7):688-695.

Keefe FJ; Caldwell DS. (1997). Cognitive behavioral control of arthritis pain. *Medicine Clinics of North America* 81(1):277-290.

Maetzel A; Ferraz MB; Bombardier C. (1998). A review of cost-effectiveness analyses in rheumatology and related disciplines. *Current Opinions in Rheumatology* 10(2):136-140.

Nicassio PM; Radojevic V; Weisman MH; Schuman C; Kim J; Schoenfeld-Smith K; Krall T. (1997). A comparison of behavioral and educational interventions for fibromyalgia. *Journal of Rheumatology* 24(10):2000-2007.

Ruof J; Hulsemann JL; Stucki G. (1999). Evaluation of costs in rheumatic diseases: A literature review. *Current Opinions in Rheumatology* 11(2):104-109.

Singh BB; Berman BM; Hadhazy VA; Creamer P. (1998). A pilot study of cognitive behavioral therapy in fibromyalgia. *Alternative Therapy Health Medicine* 4(2):67-70.

Vlaeyen JW; Teeken-Gruben NJ; Goossens ME; Rutten-van Molken MP; Pelt RA; van Eek H; Heuts PH. (1996). Cognitive-educational treatment of fibromyalgia: A randomized clinical trial. I. Clinical effects. *Journal of Rheumatology* 23(7):1237-1245.

*Cognitive Function*

Grace GM; Nielson WR; Hopkins M; Berg MA. (1999). Concentration and memory deficits in patients with fibromyalgia syndrome. *Journal of Clinical Experimental Neuropsychology* 21(4):477-487.

Landro NI; Stiles TC; Sletvold H. (1997). Memory functioning in patients with primary fibromyalgia and major depression and healthy controls. *Journal of Psychosomatic Research* 42(3):297-306.

## Collagen

Malleson P. (1998). Collagen crosslinks in fibromyalgia: Comment on the article by Sprott et al [letter; comment] *Arthritis and Rheumatism* 41(5):948-949.

Sprott H; Muller A. (1998). Collagen crosslinks as markers of a therapy effect in fibromyalgia. *Clinical Experimental Rheumatology* 16(5):626-627.

Sprott H; Muller A; Heine H. (1997). Collagen crosslinks in fibromyalgia. *Arthritis and Rheumatism* 40(8):1450-1454.

Sprott H; Muller A; Heine H. (1998). Collagen cross-links in fibromyalgia syndrome. *Zeitschrift Rheumatologie* 57 (Suppl. 2):52-55.

## Coping

Akkasilpa S; Minor M; Goldman D; Magder LS; Petri M. (2000). Association of coping responses with fibromyalgia tender points in patients with systemic lupus erythematosus. *Journal of Rheumatology* 27(3):671-674.

Buckelew SP; Huyser B; Hewett JE; Parker JC; Johnson JC; Conway R; Kay DR. (1996). Self-efficacy predicting outcome among fibromyalgia subjects. *Arthritis Care Research* 9(2):97-104.

Hellstrom O; Bullington J; Karlsson G; Lindqvist P; Mattsson B. (1999). A phenomonological study of fibromyalgia. Patient perspectives. *Scandinavian Journal of Primary Health Care* 17(1):11-16.

Jensen MP; Nielson WR; Romano JM; Hill ML; Turner JA. (2000). Further evaluation of the pain stages of change questionnaire: Is the transtheoretical model of change useful for patients with chronic pain? *Pain* 86(3):255-264.

Kelley P; Clifford P. (1997). Coping with chronic pain: Assessing narrative approaches. *Social Work* 42(3):266-277.

Martin MY; Bradley LA; Alexander RW; Alarcon GS; Triana-Alexander M; Aaron LA; Alberts KR. (1996). Coping strategies predict disability in patients with primary fibromyalgia. *Pain* 68(1):45-53.

Savelkoul M; Post MW; de Witte LP; van den Borne HB. (2000). Social support, coping and subjective well-being in patients with rheumatic diseases. *Patient Education and Counseling* 39(2-3):205-18.

Schanberg LE; Keefe FJ; Lefebvre JC; Kredich DW; Gil KM. (1996). Pain coping strategies in children with juvenile primary fibromyalgia syndrome: Correlation with pain, physical function, and psychological distress. *Arthritis Care Research* 9(2):89-96.

Schanberg LE; Keefe FJ; Lefebvre JC; Kredich DW; Gil KM. (1998). Social context of pain in children with juvenile primary fibromyalgia syndrome: Parental pain history and family environment. *Clinical Journal of Pain* 14(2):107-115.

## Copper

Biasi G; Badii F; Magaldi M; Moltoni L; Marcolongo R. (1999). [A new approach to the treatment of fibromyalgia syndrome. The use of Telo Cypro] Un nuovo approccio al trattamento della sindrome fibromialgica. L'uso del Telo Cypro. *Minerva Medica* 90(1-2):39-43.

## Cortisol

Heim C; Ehlert U; Hellhammer DH. (2000). The potential role of hypocortisolism in the pathophysiology of stress-related bodily disorders. *Psychoneuroendocrinology* 25(1):1-35.

## Cryotherapy

Metzger D; Zwingmann C; Protz W; Jackel WH. (2000). [Whole-body cryotherapy in rehabilitation of patients with rheumatoid diseases—pilot study] Die bedeutung der ganzkorperkaltetherapie im rahmen der rehabilitation bei patienten mit rheumatischen erkrankungen—ergebnisse einer pilotstudie. *Rehabilitation* (Stuttg) 39(2):93-100.

## Debrisoquine/Sparteine Polymorphism

Liska DJ. (1998). The detoxification enzyme systems. *Alternative Medicine Reviews* 3(3):187-198.

Skeith KJ; Hussain MS; Coutts RT; Ramos-Remus C; Avina-Zubieta JA; Russell AS. (1997). Adverse drug reactions and debrisoquine/sparteine (P450IID6) polymorphism in patients with fibromyalgia. *Clinical Rheumatology* 16(3):291-295.

## Dehydroepiandrosterone Sulphate

Dessein PH; Shipton EA; Joffe BI; Hadebe DP; Stanwix AE; Van der Merwe BA. (1999). Hyposecretion of adrenal androgens and the relation of serum adrenal steroids, serotonin and insulin-like growth factor-1 to clinical features in women with fibromyalgia. *Pain* 83(2):313-319.

## Dentistry

Avon SL. (1996). [Fibromyalgia in dentistry] La fibromyalgie en medecine dentaire. *Journal of the Canadian Dental Association* 62(11):874-876, 879-880.

Kotter I; Durk H; Saal JG; Kroiher A; Schweinsberg F. (1995). Mercury exposure from dental amalgam fillings in the etiology of primary fibromyalgia: A pilot study. *Journal of Rheumatology* 22(11):2194-2195.

Langworth S; Stromberg R. (1996). A case of high mercury exposure from dental amalgam. *European Journal of Oral Sciences* 104(3):320-321.

Malt UF; Nerdrum P; Oppedal B; Gundersen R; Holte M; Lone J. (1997). Physical and mental problems attributed to dental amalgam fillings: A descriptive study of 99 self-referred patients compared with 272 controls. *Psychosomatic Medicine* 59(1):32-41.

## Depression

Kurtze N; Gundersen KT; Svebak S. (1998). The role of anxiety and depression in fatigue and patterns of pain among subgroups of fibromyalgia patients. *British Journal of Medical Psychology* 71(Pt. 2):185-194.

Kurtze N; Gundersen KT; Svebak S. (1999). Quality of life, functional disability and lifestyle among subgroups of fibromyalgia patients: The significance of anxiety and depression. *British Journal of Medical Psychology* 72(Pt. 4):471-484.

Meyer-Lindenberg A; Gallhofer B. (1998). Somatized depression as a subgroup of fibromyalgia syndrome. *Zeitschrift Rheumatologie* 57 (Suppl. 2):92-93.

Morriss RK; Ahmed M; Wearden AJ; Mullis R; Strickland P; Appleby L; Campbell IT; Pearson D. (1999). The role of depression in pain, psychophysiological syndromes and medically unexplained symptoms associated with chronic fatigue syndrome. *Journal of Affective Disorders* 55(2-3):143-148.

Offenbaecher M; Glatzeder K; Ackenheil M. (1998). Self-reported depression, familial history of depression and fibromyalgia (FM), and psychological distress in patients with FM. *Zeitschrift Rheumatologie* 57 (Suppl. 2):94-96.

Okifuji A; Turk DC; Sherman JJ. (2000). Evaluation of the relationship between depression and fibromyalgia syndrome: Why aren't all patients depressed? *Journal of Rheumatology* 27(1):212-219.

Wacker HR. (2000). [Epidemiology and comorbidity of depressive disorders] Epidemiologie und komorbiditat von depressionen. *Ther Umsch* 57(2):53-58.

## Disability and Functional Impairment

Bakker C; van der Linden S; van Santen-Hoeufft M; Bolwijn P; Hidding A. (1995). Problem elicitation to assess patient priorities in ankylosing spondylitis and fibromyalgia. *Journal of Rheumatology* 22(7):1304-1310.

Beger CS. (1997). The importance of subjective claims management. *Benefits Quarterly* 13(4):41-45.

Bellamy N; Muirden KD; Brooks PM; Barraclough D; Tellus MM; Campbell J. (1999). A survey of outcome measurement procedures in routine rheumatology outpatient practice in Australia. *Journal of Rheumatology* 26(7):1593-1599.

Bennett RM. (1996). Fibromyalgia and the disability dilemma. A new era in understanding a complex, multidimensional pain syndrome. *Arthritis and Rheumatism* 39(10):1627-1634.

Blackmore MG; Gladman DD; Husted J; Long JA; Farewell VT. (1995). Measuring health status in psoriatic arthritis: The Health Assessment Questionnaire and its modification. *Journal of Rheumatology* 22(5):886-893.

Bombardier CH; Buchwald D. (1996). Chronic fatigue, chronic fatigue syndrome, and fibromyalgia. Disability and health-care use. *Medical Care* 34(9):924-930.

Buchwald D; Pearlman T; Umali J; Schmaling K; Katon W. (1996). Functional status in patients with chronic fatigue syndrome, other fatiguing illnesses, and healthy individuals. *American Journal of Medicine* 101(4):364-370.

Burckhardt CS; Bjelle A. (1996). Perceived control: A comparison of women with fibromyalgia, rheumatoid arthritis, and systemic lupus erythematosus using a Swedish version of the Rheumatology Attitudes Index. *Scandinavian Journal of Rheumatology* 25(5):300-306.

Buskila D; Neumann L. (1996). Assessing functional disability and health status of women with fibromyalgia: Validation of a Hebrew version of the Fibromyalgia Impact Questionnaire. *Journal of Rheumatology* 23(5):903-906.

Capen K. (1995). The courts, expert witnesses and fibromyalgia. *Canadian Medical Association Journal* 153(2):206-208.

Cohen ML; Quintner JL. (1998). Fibromyalgia syndrome and disability: A failed construct fails those in pain. *Medical Journal of Australia* 168(8):402-404.

Crook J; Moldofsky H; Shannon H. (1998). Determinants of disability after a work related musculoskeletal injury. *Journal of Rheumatology* 25(8):1570-1577.

Department of Veterans Affairs (VA). (1999). Schedule for rating disabilities: Fibromyalgia. Final rule. *Federal Registry* 64(116):32410-32411.

Duro JC. (1997). Fibromyalgia and disability. *Journal of Rheumatology* 24(1):229; discussion 230-231.

Escalante A; Galarza-Delgado D; Beardmore TD; Baethge BA; Esquivel-Valerio J; Marines AL; Mingrone M. (1996). Cross-cultural adaptation of a brief outcome questionnaire for Spanish-speaking arthritis patients. *Arthritis and Rheumatism* 39(1):93-100.

Fibromyalgia syndrome. Feeling more pain. (1999). *Harvard Health Letters* 24(12):4-5.

Friedman PJ. (1997). Predictors of work disability in work-related upper-extremity disorders. *Journal of Occupational and Environmental Medicine* 39(4):339-343.

Gjesdal S; Kristiansen AM. (1997). [Norwegian fibromyalgia epidemic—its rise or possible decline. What is the trend based on disability statistics?] Den norske fibromyalgi-epidemiens vekst—og mulige fall. Hva viser uforestatistikken? *Tidsskr Nor Laegeforen* 117(17):2449-2453.

Goldenberg DL; Mossey CJ; Schmid CH. (1995). A model to assess severity and impact of fibromyalgia. *Journal of Rheumatology* 22(12):2313-2318.

Goossens ME; Vlaeyen JW; Rutten-van Molken MP; van der Linden SM. (1999). Patient utilities in chronic musculoskeletal pain: How useful is the standard gamble method? *Pain* 80(1-2):365-375.

Gordon DA. (1999). Chronic widespread pain as a medico-legal issue. *Baillieres Best Practice Research in Clinical Rheumatology* 13(3):531-543.

Helfenstein M; Feldman D. (2000). The pervasiveness of the illness suffered by workers seeking compensation for disabling arm pain. *Journal of Occupational and Environmental Medicine* 42(2):171-175.

Henriksson C; Burckhardt C. (1996). Impact of fibromyalgia on everyday life: A study of women in the USA and Sweden. *Disability and Rehabilitation* 18(5):241-248.

Henriksson C; Liedberg G. (2000). Factors of importance for work disability in women with fibromyalgia. *Journal of Rheumatology* 27(5):1271-1276.

Huber M. (2000). [Aspects of occupational disability in psychosomatic disorders] Aspekte der berufsunfahigkeit bei psychosomatischen erkrankungen. *Versicherungsmedizin* 52(2):66-75.

Huston GJ. (2000). A fibromyalgia scale in a general rheumatology clinic. *Rheumatology* (Oxford) 39(3):336-337.

Jason LA; Taylor RR; Kennedy CL. (2000). Chronic fatigue syndrome, fibromyalgia, and multiple chemical sensitivities in a community-based sample of persons with chronic fatigue syndrome-like symptoms. *Psychosomatic Medicine* 62(5):655-663.

Kaplan RM; Schmidt SM; Cronan TA. (2000). Quality of well-being in patients with fibromyalgia. *Journal of Rheumatology* 27(3):785-789.

Keitel W. (1999). [Fibromyalgia syndrome—out of control?] Das fibromyalgie-syndrom—ausser kontrolle? *Fortschrift Medizin* 117(5):32-36.

King S; Wessel J; Bhambhani Y; Maikala R; Sholter D; Maksymowych W. (1999). Validity and reliability of the 6-minute walk in persons with fibromyalgia. *Journal of Rheumatology* 26(10):2233-2237.

Kovarsky J. (1997). Which physicians are qualified to evaluate disability in fibromyalgia? Comment on the article by Bennett. *Arthritis and Rheumatism* 40(6):1184-1185.

Krapac L; Sladoljev M; Sacer D; Sakic D. (1997). Rheumatic complaints and musculoskeletal disorders in workers of a meat processing industry. *Arh Hig Rada Toksikol* 48(2):211-217.

Littlejohn GO. (1998). Fibromyalgia syndrome and disability: The neurogenic model. *Medical Journal of Australia* 168(8):398-401.

Long JA; Husted JA; Gladman DD; Farewell VT. (2000). The relationship between patient satisfaction with health and clinical measures of function and disease status in patients with psoriatic arthritis. *Journal of Rheumatology* 27(4):958-966.

Lousberg R; Van Breukelen GJ; Groenman NH; Schmidt AJ; Arntz A; Winter FA. (1999). Psychometric properties of the Multidimensional Pain Inventory, Dutch language version (MPI-DLV). *Behavioral Research Therapy* 37(2):167-182.

Mailis A; Furlong W; Taylor A. (2000). Chronic pain in a family of 6 in the context of litigation. *Journal of Rheumatology* 27(5):1315-1317.

Malterud K. (1999). ["Uncertain" health complaints of women—a challenge for medicine and welfare state policy] Kvinners "ubestemte" helseplager—medisinske og velferdspolitiske utfordringer. *Tidsskr Nor Laegeforen* 119(12):1790-1793.

Mannerkorpi K; Ekdahl C. (1997). Assessment of functional limitation and disability in patients with fibromyalgia. *Scandinavian Journal of Rheumatology* 26(1):4-13.

Mannerkorpi K; Svantesson U; Carlsson J; Ekdahl C. (1999). Tests of functional limitations in fibromyalgia syndrome: A reliability study. *Arthritis Care Research* 12(3):193-199.

Martin MY; Bradley LA; Alexander RW; Alarcon GS; Triana-Alexander M; Aaron LA; Alberts KR. (1996). Coping strategies predict disability in patients with primary fibromyalgia. *Pain* 68(1):45-53.

Neumann L; Berzak A; Buskila D. (2000). Measuring health status in Israeli patients with fibromyalgia syndrome and widespread pain and healthy individuals: Utility of the short form 36-item health survey (SF-36). *Seminars in Arthritis and Rheumatism* 29(6):400-408.

Neumann L; Dudnik Y; Bolotin A; Buskila D. (1999). Evaluation of a Hebrew version of the revised and expanded Arthritis Impact Measurement Scales (AIMS2) in patients with fibromyalgia. *Journal of Rheumatology* 26(8):1816-1821.

Neumann L; Press J; Glibitzki M; Bolotin A; Rubinow A; Buskila D. (2000). CLINHAQ scale—validation of a Hebrew version in patients with fibromyalgia. Clinical Health Assessment Questionnaire. *Clinical Rheumatology* 19(4):265-269.

Nordenskiold U. (1997). Daily activities in women with rheumatoid arthritis. Aspects of patient education, assistive devices and methods for disability and impairment assessment. *Scandinavian Journal of Rehabilitative Medicine* (Suppl. 37):1-72.

Offenbaecher M; Waltz M; Schoeps P. (2000). Validation of a German version of the Fibromyalgia Impact Questionnaire (FIQ-G). *Journal of Rheumatology* 27(8):1984-1988.

Ortiz Z; Shea B; Garcia Dieguez M; Boers M; Tugwell P; Boonen A; Wells G. (1999). The responsiveness of generic quality of life instruments in rheumatic diseases. A systematic review of randomized controlled trials. *Journal of Rheumatology* 26(1):210-216.

Pellegrino MJ; Waylonis GW. (1997). Fibromyalgia and disability. *Journal of Rheumatology* 24(1):229-230; discussion 230-231.

Pincus T; Swearingen C; Wolfe F. (1999). Toward a multidimensional Health Assessment Questionnaire (MDHAQ): Assessment of advanced activities of daily living and psychological status in the patient-friendly health assessment questionnaire format. *Arthritis and Rheumatism* 42(10):2220-2230.

Rocca PV. (1999). Fibromyalgia: How disabling? *Delaware Medical Journal* 71(6):263-265.

Smith MD. (1997). Fibromyalgia and disability. *Journal of Rheumatology* 24(1):229; discussion 230-231.

Soderberg S; Lundman B; Norberg A. (1999). Struggling for dignity: The meaning of women's experiences of living with fibromyalgia. *Quality Health Research* 9(5):575-587.

Turk DC; Okifuji A; Starz TW; Sinclair JD. (1996). Effects of type of symptom onset on psychological distress and disability in fibromyalgia syndrome patients. *Pain* 68(2-3):423-430.

Van Linthoudt D; Ferrari R; Babaiantz O; Ott H. (2000). [Rheumatology expertise] Expertises rhumatologiques. *Revue Medicale Suisse Romande* 120(1):73-80.

White KP; Harth M; Teasell RW. (1995). Work disability evaluation and the fibromyalgia syndrome. *Seminars in Arthritis and Rheumatism* 24(6):371-381.

White KP; Speechley M; Harth M; Ostbye T. (1999). Comparing self-reported function and work disability in 100 community cases of fibromyalgia syndrome versus controls in London, Ontario: The London Fibromyalgia Epidemiology Study. *Arthritis and Rheumatism* 42(1):76-83.

Wigers SH. (1996). Fibromyalgia outcome: The predictive values of symptom duration, physical activity, disability pension, and critical life events—a 4.5 year prospective study. *Journal of Psychosomatic Research* 41(3):235-243.

Wolfe F. (1996). The fibromyalgia syndrome: A consensus report on fibromyalgia and disability. *Journal of Rheumatology* 23(3):534-539.

Wolfe F. (1999). Determinants of WOMAC function, pain and stiffness scores: Evidence for the role of low back pain, symptom counts, fatigue and depression in osteoarthritis, rheumatoid arthritis and fibromyalgia. *Rheumatology* (Oxford) 38(4):355-361.

Wolfe F. (2000). For example is not evidence: Fibromyalgia and the law. *Journal of Rheumatology* 27(5):1115-1116.

Wolfe F; Anderson J; Harkness D; Bennett RM; Caro XJ; Goldenberg DL; Russell IJ; Yunus MB. (1997a). Health status and disease severity in fibromyalgia: results of a six-center longitudinal study. *Arthritis and Rheumatism* 40(9):1571-1579.

Wolfe F; Anderson J; Harkness D; Bennett RM; Caro XJ; Goldenberg DL; Russell IJ; Yunus MB. (1997b). Work and disability status of persons with fibromyalgia. *Journal of Rheumatology* 24(6):1171-1178.

Wolfe F; Hawley DJ. (1999). Evidence of disordered symptom appraisal in fibromyalgia: Increased rates of reported comorbidity and comorbidity severity. *Clinical and Experimental Rheumatology* 17(3):297-303.

Wolfe F; Hawley DJ; Goldenberg DL; Russell IJ; Buskila D; Neumann L. (2000). The assessment of functional impairment in fibromyalgia (FM): Rasch analyses of 5 functional scales and the development of the FM Health Assessment Questionnaire. *Journal of Rheumatology* 27(8):1989-1999.

Wolfe F; Kong SX. (1999). Rasch analysis of the Western Ontario MacMaster questionnaire (WOMAC) in 2205 patients with osteoarthritis, rheumatoid arthritis, and fibromyalgia. *Annals of Rheumatic Diseases* 58(9):563-568.

Wolfe F; Potter J. (1996). Fibromyalgia and work disability: Is Fibromyalgia a disabling disorder? *Rheumatic Disease Clinics of North America* 22(2):369-391.

Worz R. (1999). [Fibromyalgia—a current challenge. Considerations for insurance and social security dimensions] Fibromyalgie—eine herausforderung unserer zeit. beachtenswerte versicherungs- und sozialrechtliche dimension. *Fortschrift Medizin* 117(5):37.

*Dizziness*

Rusy LM; Harvey SA; Beste DJ. (1999). Pediatric fibromyalgia and dizziness: Evaluation of vestibular function. *Journal of Developmental Behavioral Pediatrics* 20(4):211-215.

*Effort*

Norregaard J; Bulow PM; Lykkegaard JJ; Mehlsen J; Danneskiold-Samsooe B. (1997). Muscle strength, working capacity and effort in patients with fibromyalgia. *Scandinavian Journal of Rehabilitative Medicine* 29(2):97-102.

*Ehlers-Danlos Syndrome*

Miller VJ; Zeltser R; Yoeli Z; Bodner L. (1997). Ehlers-Danlos syndrome, fibromyalgia and temporomandibular disorder: Report of an unusual combination. *Cranio* 15(3):267-269.

*Eosinophilia-Myalgia Syndrome*

Barth H; Berg PA; Klein R. (1999). Is there any relationship between eosinophilia myalgia syndrome (EMS) and fibromyalgia syndrome (FMS)? An analysis of clinical and immunological data. *Advances in Experimental Medical Biology* 467:487-496.

Hudson JI; Pope HG Jr; Carter WP; Daniels SR. (1996). Fibromyalgia, psychiatric disorders, and assessment of the longterm outcome of eosinophilia-myalgia syndrome. *Journal of Rheumatology* (Suppl. 46):37-42; discussion 42-43.

Taylor RM; Gabriel SE; O'Fallon WM; Bowles CA; Duffy J. (1996). A diagnostic algorithm for distinguishing the eosinophilia-myalgia syndrome from fibromyalgia and chronic myofascial pain. *Journal of Rheumatology* (Suppl. 46):13-18.

*Epidemiology*

Bazelmans E; Vercoulen JH; Galama JM; van Weel C; van der Meer JW; Bleijenberg G. (1997). [Prevalence of chronic fatigue syndrome and primary fibromyalgia syndrome in The Netherlands (published erratum appears in *Ned Tijdschr Geneeskd* 1997, September 13;141(37):2686)] Prevalentie van het chronische-vermoeidheidsyndroom en het primaire-fibromyalgiesyndroom in Nederland. *Ned Tijdschr Geneeskd* 141(31):1520-1523.

Bellamy N; Kaloni S; Pope J; Coulter K; Campbell J. (1998). Quantitative rheumatology: A survey of outcome measurement procedures in routine rheumatology outpatient practice in Canada. *Journal of Rheumatology* 25(5):852-858.

Clark P; Burgos-Vargas R; Medina-Palma C; Lavielle P; Marina FF. (1998). Prevalence of fibromyalgia in children: A clinical study of Mexican children. *Journal of Rheumatology* 25(10):2009-2014.

Farooqi A; Gibson T. (1998). Prevalence of the major rheumatic disorders in the adult population of north Pakistan. *British Journal of Rheumatology* 37(5):491-495.

Forseth KO. (1997). [The Norwegian fibromyalgia epidemics' growth—and possible decline] Den norske fibromyalgi-epidemiens vekstog mulige fall. *Tidsskr Nor Laegeforen* 117(20):2999-3000.

Forseth KO; Gran JT; Husby G. (1997). A population study of the incidence of fibromyalgia among women aged 26-55 yr. *British Journal of Rheumatology* 36(12):1318-1323.

Gare BA. (1996). Epidemiology of rheumatic disease in children. *Current Opinions in Rheumatology* 8(5):449-454.

Goldenberg DL. (1996). Fibromyalgia, chronic fatigue syndrome, and myofascial pain. *Current Opinions in Rheumatology* 8(2):113-123.

Gordon S; Morrison C. (1998). Fibromyalgia and its primary care implications. *Medsurg Nursing* 7(4):207-213, 216.

Gran JT; Nordvag BY. (2000). [Referrals from general practitioners to rheumatologists] Henvisninger fra primaerleger til revmatologisk poliklinikk. *Tidsskr Nor Laegeforen* 120(13):1529-1532.

Jacobsson LT; Nagi DK; Pillemer SR; Knowler WC; Hanson RL; Pettitt DJ; Bennett PH. (1996). Low prevalences of chronic widespread pain and shoulder disorders among the Pima Indians. *Journal of Rheumatology* 23(5):907-909.

Jason LA; Taylor RR; Kennedy CL. (2000). Chronic fatigue syndrome, fibromyalgia, and multiple chemical sensitivities in a community-based sample of persons with chronic fatigue syndrome-like symptoms. *Psychosomatic Medicine* 62(5):655-663.

Karaaslan Y; Ozturk M; Haznedaroglu S. (1999). Secondary fibromyalgia in Turkish patients with rheumatologic disorders. *Lupus* 8(6):486.

Lawrence RC; Helmick CG; Arnett FC; Deyo RA; Felson DT; Giannini EH; Heyse SP; Hirsch R; Hochberg MC; Hunder GG; Liang MH; Pillemer SR; Steen VD; Wolfe F. (1998). Estimates of the prevalence of arthritis and selected musculoskeletal disorders in the United States. *Arthritis and Rheumatism* 41(5):778-799.

Linaker CH; Walker-Bone K; Palmer K; Cooper C. (1999). Frequency and impact of regional musculoskeletal disorders. *Baillieres Best Practice Research in Clinical Rheumatology* 13(2):197-215.

Sardini S; Ghirardini M; Betelemme L; Arpino C; Fatti F; Zanini F. (1996). [Epidemiological study of a primary fibromyalgia in pediatric age] Studio epidemiologico sulla fibromialgia primaria in eta pediatrica. *Minerva Pediatrica* 48(12):543-550.

Smith WA. (1998). Fibromyalgia syndrome. *Nursing Clinics of North America* 33(4):653-669.
White KP; Harth M; Speechley M; Ostbye T. (1999). Testing an instrument to screen for fibromyalgia syndrome in general population studies: The London Fibromyalgia Epidemiology Study Screening Questionnaire. *Journal of Rheumatology* 26(4):880-884.
White KP; Speechley M; Harth M; Ostbye T. (1999a). The London Fibromyalgia Epidemiology Study: Comparing the demographic and clinical characteristics in 100 random community cases of fibromyalgia versus controls. *Journal of Rheumatology* 26(7):1577-1585.
White KP; Speechley M; Harth M; Ostbye T. (1999b). The London Fibromyalgia Epidemiology Study: Direct health care costs of fibromyalgia syndrome in London, Canada. *Journal of Rheumatology* 26(4):885-889.
White KP; Speechley M; Harth M; Ostbye T. (1999c). The London Fibromyalgia Epidemiology Study: The prevalence of fibromyalgia syndrome in London, Ontario. *Journal of Rheumatology* 26(7):1570-1576.

## *Epstein-Barr Virus*

McCarty DJ; Csuka ME. (1998). Polysynovitis associated with acute Epstein-Barr virus infection. *Journal of Rheumatology* 25(10):2039-2040.

## **Erb** *Gene*

Lowe JC; Cullum ME; Graf LH Jr; Yellin J. (1997). Mutations in the c-erbA beta 1 gene: Do they underlie euthyroid fibromyalgia? *Medical Hypotheses* 48(2):125-135.

## *Ergonomics*

Kreczy A; Kofler M; Gschwendtner A. (1999). Underestimated health hazard: Proposal for an ergonomic microscope workstation. *Lancet* 354(9191):1701-1702.
Van Houdenhove B; Neerinckx E. (1999). Is "ergomania" a predisposing factor to chronic pain and fatigue? *Psychosomatics* 40(6):529-530.

## *Erythrocyte Sedimentation Rate*

Suarez-Almazor ME; Gonzalez-Lopez L; Gamez-Nava JI; Belseck E; Kendall CJ; Davis P. (1998). Utilization and predictive value of laboratory tests in patients referred to rheumatologists by primary care physicians. *Journal of Rheumatology* 25(10):1980-1985.

**Exercise**

Buckelew SP; Conway R; Parker J; Deuser WE; Read J; Witty TE; Hewett JE; Minor M; Johnson JC; Van Male L; McIntosh MJ; Nigh M; Kay DR. (1998). Biofeedback/relaxation training and exercise interventions for fibromyalgia: A prospective trial. *Arthritis Care Research* 11(3):196-209.

Deuster PA. (1996). Exercise in the prevention and treatment of chronic disorders. *Women's Health Issues* 6(6):320-331.

Dominick KL; Gullette EC; Babyak MA; Mallow KL; Sherwood A; Waugh R; Chilikuri M; Keefe FJ; Blumenthal JA. (1999). Predicting peak oxygen uptake among older patients with chronic illness. *Journal of Cardiopulmonary Rehabilitation* 19(2):81-89.

Gowans SE; deHueck A; Voss S; Richardson M. (1999). A randomized, controlled trial of exercise and education for individuals with fibromyalgia. *Arthritis Care Research* 12(2):120-128.

Han SS. (1998). [Effects of a self-help program including stretching exercise on symptom reduction in patients with fibromyalgia] *Taehan Kanho* 37(1):78-80.

Mannerkorpi K; Nyberg B; Ahlmen M; Ekdahl C. (2000). Pool exercise combined with an education program for patients with fibromyalgia syndrome. A prospective, randomized study. *Journal of Rheumatology* 27(10):2473-2481.

Martin L; Nutting A; MacIntosh BR; Edworthy SM; Butterwick D; Cook J. (1996). An exercise program in the treatment of fibromyalgia. *Journal of Rheumatology* 23(6):1050-1053.

Meiworm L; Jakob E; Walker UA; Peter HH; Keul J. (2000). Patients with fibromyalgia benefit from aerobic endurance exercise. *Clinical Rheumatology* 19(4): 253-257.

Mengshoel AM. (1996). [Effect of physical exercise in fibromyalgia] Effekt av fysisk trening ved fibromyalgi. *Tidsskr Nor Laegeforen* 116(6):746-748.

Mengshoel AM; Vollestad NK; Forre O. (1995). Pain and fatigue induced by exercise in fibromyalgia patients and sedentary healthy subjects. *Clinical and Experimental Rheumatology* 13(4):477-482.

Meyer BB; Lemley KJ. (2000). Utilizing exercise to affect the symptomology of fibromyalgia: A pilot study. *Medical Science Sports Exercise* 32(10):1691-1697.

Ramsay C; Moreland J; Ho M; Joyce S; Walker S; Pullar T. (2000). An observer-blinded comparison of supervised and unsupervised aerobic exercise regimens in fibromyalgia. *Rheumatology* (Oxford) 39(5):501-505.

Wigers SH; Stiles TC; Vogel PA. (1996). Effects of aerobic exercise versus stress management treatment in fibromyalgia. A 4.5 year prospective study. *Scandinavian Journal of Rheumatology* 25(2):77-86.

*Fatigue*

Groopman JE. (1998). Fatigue in cancer and HIV/AIDS. *Oncology* 12(3):335-344.

Llewelyn MB. (1996). Assessing the fatigued patient. *British Journal of Hospital Medicine* 55(3):125-129.

Miller TA; Allen GM; Gandevia SC. (1996). Muscle force, perceived effort, and voluntary activation of the elbow flexors assessed with sensitive twitch interpolation in fibromyalgia. *Journal of Rheumatology* 23(9):1621-1627.

Ream E; Richardson A. (1996). Fatigue: A concept analysis. *International Journal of Nursing Studies* 33(5):519-529.

Shapiro CM. (1998). Fatigue: How many types and how common? *Journal of Psychosomatic Research* 45:1-3.

Tiesinga LJ; Dassen TW; Halfens RJ. (1996). Fatigue: A summary of the definitions, dimensions, and indicators. *Nursing Diagnosis* 7(2):51-62.

Ward MH; DeLisle H; Shores JH; Slocum PC; Foresman BH. (1996). Chronic fatigue complaints in primary care: Incidence and diagnostic patterns. *Journal of the American Osteopathic Association* 96(1):34-46, 41.

White PD. (1997). The relationship between infection and fatigue. *Journal of Psychosomatic Research* 43(4):345-350.

Wolfe F; Hawley DJ; Wilson K. (1996). The prevalence and meaning of fatigue in rheumatic disease. *Journal of Rheumatology* 23(8):1407-1417.

*Fibromyalgia*

Affleck G; Tennen H; Urrows S; Higgins P; Abeles M; Hall C; Karoly P; Newton C. (1998). Fibromyalgia and women's pursuit of personal goals: A daily process analysis. *Health and Psychology* 17(1):40-47.

Alarcon GS. (1997). Arthralgias, myalgias, facial erythema, and a positive ANA: Not necessarily SLE. *Cleveland Clinic Journal of Medicine* 64(7):361-364.

Ang D; Wilke WS. (1999). Diagnosis, etiology, and therapy of fibromyalgia. *Comprehensive Therapy* 25(4):221-227.

Armstrong R. (2000). Fibromyalgia: Is recovery impeded by the internet? *Archives of Internal Medicine* 160(7):1039-1040.

Asencio-Marchante JJ; Terriza-Garcia F. (1998). [Myalgia-fasciculation syndrome] Sindrome de mialgia-fasciculacion. *Revista Neurologica* 26(149):162.

Barth WF. (1997). Office evaluation of the patient with musculoskeletal complaints. *American Journal of Medicine* 102(1A):3S-10S.

Baschetti R. (1999). Fibromyalgia, chronic fatigue syndrome, and Addison disease. *Archives of Internal Medicine* 159(20):2481; discussion 2482-2483.

Bassetti S. (1996). [A case from practice. Fibromyalgia] Der fall aus der prazis (352). Fibromyalgie. *Schweize Rundschrift Medizin Prax* 85(22):730-731.

Bazelmans E; Vercoulen JH; Galama JM; van Weel C; van der Meer JW; Bleijenberg G. (1997). Prevalence of chronic fatigue syndrome and primary fibromyalgia syndrome in the Netherlands. *Nederlands Tijdschrift voor Geneeskunde* 141(31):1520-1523.

Bennett R. (1998). Fibromyalgia, chronic fatigue syndrome, and myofascial pain. *Current Opinions in Rheumatology* 10(2):95-103.

Ben-Zion I; Shieber A; Buskila D. (1996). Psychiatric aspects of fibromyalgia syndrome. *Harefuah* 131(3-4):127-129.

Borenstein D. (1996). Epidemiology, etiology, diagnostic evaluation, and treatment of low back pain. *Current Opinions in Rheumatology* 8(2):124-129.

Briggs FE. (1997). Fibromyalgia: An important diagnosis to consider. *Nurse Practice* 22(8):27-28.

Brown CR. (1997). Fibromyalgia. *Practice Periodontics and Aesthetic Dentistry* 9(8):878, 883.

Buchwald D. (1996). Fibromyalgia and chronic fatigue syndrome: Similarities and differences. *Rheumatic Diseases Clinics of North America* 22(2):219-243.

Buskila D. (1999). Fibromyalgia, chronic fatigue syndrome, and myofascial pain syndrome. *Current Opinions in Rheumatology* 11(2):119-126.

Buskila D. (2000). Fibromyalgia, chronic fatigue syndrome, and myofascial pain syndrome. *Current Opinions in Rheumatology* 12(2):113-123.

Buskila D; Neumann L; Sibirski D; Shvartzman P. (1997). Awareness of diagnostic and clinical features of fibromyalgia among family physicians. *Family Practice* 14(3):238-241.

Cathebras P. (1997). [What is a disease?] Qu'est-ce qu'une maladie? *Revue Medicine Interne* 18(10):809-813.

Cathebras P. (2000). [Should fibromyalgia survive the century?] La fibromyalgie doit-elle passer le siecle? *Revue Medicale Interne* 21(7):577-579.

Cathebras P; Lauwers A; Rousset H. (1998). [Fibromyalgia. A critical review] La fibromyalgie. Une revue critique. *Annales Medicine Interne* (Paris) 149(7):406-414.

Celiker R; Borman P; Oktem F; Gokce-Kutsal Y; Basgoze O. (1997). Psychological disturbance in fibromyalgia: Relation to pain severity. *Clinical Rheumatology* 16(2):179-184.

Chambers CR. (1997). Fireworks over fibromyalgia, CFS, and IBS. *Postgraduate Medicine* 102(6):43.

Cherin P; Authier FJ; Gherardi RK; Romero N; Laforet P; Eymard B; Herson S; Caillat-Vigneron N. (2000). Gallium-67 scintigraphy in macrophagic myofasciitis. *Arthritis and Rheumatism* 43(7):1520-1526.

Clauw DJ. (1995). Fibromyalgia: More than just a musculoskeletal disease. *American Family Physician* 52(3):843-51, 853-854.

Cohen ML. (1999). Is fibromyalgia a distinct clinical entity? The disapproving rheumatologist's evidence. *Baillieres Best Practice Research in Clinical Rheumatology* 13(3):421-425.

Coward BL. (1999). Clinical snapshot. Fibromyalgia. *American Journal of Nursing* 99(10):42-43.

Csef H. (1999). [Similarities of chronic fatigue syndrome, fibromyalgia and multiple chemical sensitivity] Gemeinsamkeiten von chronic fatigue syndrom, fibromyalgie und multipler chemischer sensitivitat. *Deutsche Medizin Wochenschrift* 124(6):163-169.

Cunningham ME. (1996). Becoming familiar with fibromyalgia. *Orthopedic Nursing* 15(2):33-36.

de Jesus M. (2000). Fibromyalgia onset. *American Journal of Nursing* 100(1):14.

Fibromyalgia. (2000). *Health News* 6(2):1-2.

Fibromyalgia Syndrome—An interdisciplinary challenge of basic and clinical science. International conference. Bad Nauheim, Germany, October 23-25, (1997). Abstracts. *Zeitschrift Rheumatologie* 56(6):351-379.

Finestone AJ. (1997). A doctor's dilemma. Is a diagnosis disabling or enabling? *Archives of Internal Medicine* 157(5):491-492.

Fitzcharles MA. (1999). Is fibromyalgia a distinct clinical entity? The approving rheumatologist's evidence. *Baillieres Best Practice Research in Clinical Rheumatology* 13(3):437-443.

Fitzcharles MA; Esdaile JM. (1997). The overdiagnosis of fibromyalgia syndrome. *American Journal of Medicine* 103(1):44-50.

Fordyce WE. (2000). Fibromyalgia and related matters. *Clinical Journal of Pain* 16(2):181-182.

Gamez-Nava JI; Gonzalez-Lopez L; Davis P; Suarez-Almazor ME. (1998). Referral and diagnosis of common rheumatic diseases by primary care physicians. *British Journal of Rheumatology* 37(11):1215-1219.

Garfin SR. (1995). A 50-year-old woman with disabling spinal stenosis. *Journal of the American Medical Association* 274(24):1949-1954.

Gelfand SG. (1998). Fibromyalgia: More questions and implications. *Arthritis and Rheumatism* 41(6):1138-1139.

Gerster JC. (1999). [Fibromyalgia. Past and present] Fibromyalgie. Le passe, le present. *Revue Medicale Suisse Romande* 119(6):513-516.

Goldenberg DL. (1996). What is the future of fibromyalgia? *Rheumatic Diseases Clinics of North America* 22(2):393-406.

Goldenberg DL. (1997). Fibromyalgia, chronic fatigue syndrome, and myofascial pain syndrome. *Current Opinions in Rheumatology* 9(2):135-143.

Goldenberg DL. (1999). Fibromyalgia syndrome a decade later: What have we learned? *Archives of Internal Medicine* 159(8):777-785.

Gordon DA. (1997). Fibromyalgia—out of control? *Journal of Rheumatology* 24(7):1247.

Gordon S; Morrison C. (1998). Fibromyalgia and its primary care implications. *Medsurg Nursing* 7(4):207-213, 216.

Grahame R. (2000). Pain, distress and joint hyperlaxity. *Joint, Bone and Spine* 67(3):157-163.

Granzow B. (1999). [Mutual features of chronic fatigue syndrome, fibromyalgia and multiple chemical sensitivity] Gemeinsamkeiten von chronic fatique syndrom, fibromyalgie und multipler chemischer sensitivitat. *Deutsche Medizin Wochenschrift* 124(41):1224.

Hadler NM. (1996a). Is fibromyalgia a useful diagnostic label? *Cleveland Clinic Journal of Medicine* 63(2):85-87.

Hadler NM. (1996b). If you have to prove you are ill, you can't get well. The object lesson of fibromyalgia. *Spine* 1521(20):2397-2400.

Hadler NM. (1997a). Fibromyalgia, chronic fatigue, and other iatrogenic diagnostic algorithms. Do some labels escalate illness in vulnerable patients? *Postgraduate Medicine* 102(2):161-162, 165-166, 171-172 passim.

Hadler NM. (1997b). Fibromyalgia: La maladie est morte. Vive le malade! *Journal of Rheumatology* 24(7):1250-1251; discussion 1252.

Hamilton SF. (1998). The fibromyalgia problem. *Journal of Rheumatology* 25(5):1027-1028; discussion 1028-1030.

Handler RP. (1998). The fibromyalgia problem. *Journal of Rheumatology* 25(5):1025; discussion 1028-1030.

Hantzschel H; Boche K. (1999). [Fibromyalgia syndrome] Das fibromyalgie-syndrom. *Fortschrift Medizin* 117(5):26-8, 30-31.

Hart FD. (1998). Underlying signs of fibromyalgia. *Practitioner* 242(1586):407-410.

Hausotter W. (1998). [Fibromyalgia—a dispensable disease term?] Fibromyalgie—ein entbehrlicher Krankheitsbegriff? *Versicherungsmedizin* 50(1):13-17.

Healey LA. (1996). On fibromyalgia. *Bulletin of Rheumatic Diseases* 45(6):1.

Helliwell PS. (1995). The semeiology of arthritis: Discriminating between patients on the basis of their symptoms. *Annals of Rheumatic Diseases* 54(11):924-926.

Hellstrom OW. (1995). Health promotion and clinical dialogue. *Patient Education Counselling* 25(3):247-256.

Hellstrom O; Bullington J; Karlsson G; Lindqvist P; Mattsson B. (1998). Doctors' attitudes to fibromyalgia: A phenomenological study. *Scandinavian Journal of Social Medicine* 26(3):232-237.

Henriksson KG. (1999). Is fibromyalgia a distinct clinical entity? Pain mechanisms in fibromyalgia syndrome. A myologist's view. *Baillieres Best Practice Research in Clinical Rheumatology* 13(3):455-461.

Hilden J. (1996). [Diagnosis of fibromyalgia. A critical review of the Scandinavian literature] Fibromyalgidiagnosen. En kritisk oversigt over nordisk litteratur. *Nordisk Medizin* 111(9):308-312.

Hoffmann A; Linder R; Kroger B; Schnabel A; Kruger GR. (1996). Fibromyalgia syndrome and chronic fatigue syndrome. Similarities and differences. *Deutsche Medizin Wochenschrift* 121(38):1165-1168.

Holland NW; Gonzalez EB. (1998). Soft tissue problems in older adults. *Clinical Geriatric Medicine* 14(3):601-611.

Holoweiko M. (1996). Holding the line on elusive ailments. *Business Health* 14(12):30-32, 35-37.

Hudson AJ. (1998). The fibromyalgia problem. *Journal of Rheumatology* 25(5): 1025-1026; discussion 1028-1030.

Hunt S; Starkebaum G; Thompson CE. (1998). The fibromyalgia problem. *Journal of Rheumatology* 25(5):1023-1024; discussion 1028-1030.

Hyams KC. (1998). Developing case definitions for symptom-based conditions: The problem of specificity. *Epidemiology Reviews* 20(2):148-156.

Jacobsen S. (2000). [Chronic musculoskeletal pain syndromes] Kroniske muskelsmertesyndromer. *Ugeskr Laeger* 162(15):2178-2180.

Jahn K; Klenke T. (1999). [Web sites on tinnitus, fibromyalgia, chronic fatigue syndrome, etc. Here your patients seek information] Webseiten uber tinnitus, fibromyalgie, mudigkeitssyndrom etc. Hier informieren sich ihre patienten. *MMW Fortschrift Medizin* 141(51-52):14.

Jones RC. (1996). Fibromyalgia: Misdiagnosed, mistreated and misunderstood? *American Family Physician* 53(1):91-92.

Kaden M; Bubenzer RH. (1999). [License fee for fibromyalgia? Illness with trademark protection] Lizenzgebuhr fur fibromyalgie? Krankheit mit markenschutz. *MMW Fortschrift Medizin* 141(46):60.

Katz JN; Barrett J; Liang MH; Bacon AM; Kaplan H; Kieval RI; Lindsey SM; Roberts WN; Sheff DM; Spencer RT; Weaver AL; Baron JA. (1997). Sensitivity and positive predictive value of Medicare Part B physician claims for rheumatologic diagnoses and procedures. *Arthritis and Rheumatism* 40(9):1594-1600.

Kavanaugh AF. (1996). Fibromyalgia or multi-organ dysesthesia? *Arthritis and Rheumatism* 39(1):180-181.

Keitel W. (1997). [Backache from the internal medicine-rheumatologic viewpoint] Ruckenschmerz aus internistisch-rheumatologischer sicht. *Zeitschrift Arztliche Fortbildung* (Jena) 90(8):671-676.

Kelemen J; Muller W. (1998). [Secondary fibromyalgia. Differentiation of primary and secondary fibromyalgia is necessary for successful therapy] Sekundare fibromyalgien. Differenzierung primarer und sekundarer fibromyalgien notwendig fur erfolgreiche therapie. *Fortschrift Medizin* 116(10):44-46.

Kelly MC. (1997). Fibromyalgia syndrome. *Irish Medical Journal* 90(1):14, 16.

Kennedy M; Felson DT. (1996). A prospective long-term study of fibromyalgia syndrome. *Arthritis and Rheumatism* 39(4):682-685.

Kenner C. (1998). Fibromyalgia and chronic fatigue: The holistic perspective. *Holistic Nursing Practice* 12(3):55-63.

Kissel W; Mahnig P. (1998). [Fibromyalgia (generalized tendomyopathy) in expert assessment. Analysis of 158 cases] Die fibromyalgie (generalisierte tendomyopathie) in der begutachtungssituation. Analyse von 158 fallen. *Schweize Rundschrift Medizin Prax* 87(16):538-545.

Kjaergaard J. (1998). [Fibromyalgia] Fibromyalgi. *Ugeskr Laeger* 160(25):3751.

Klimas N. (1998). Pathogenesis of chronic fatigue syndrome and fibromyalgia. *Growth Hormone and IGF Research* 8 (Suppl. B):123-126.

Klineberg I; McGregor N; Butt H; Dunstan H; Roberts T; Zerbes M. (1998). Chronic orofacial muscle pain: A new approach to diagnosis and management. *Alpha Omegan* 91(2):25-28.

Krsnich-Shriwise S. (1997). Fibromyalgia syndrome: An overview. *Physical Therapy* 77(1):68-75.

Kuhn P. (2000). [Fibromyalgia at the crossroads of rheumatology, psychology and social work] La fibromyalgie au carrefour de la rhumatologie, de la psychologie et des assurances sociales. *R. Darioli et J. Perdrix, RMSR*, 120: 471-474, no. 5.

Kurtze N; Gundersen KT; Svebak S. (1998). The role of anxiety and depression in fatigue and patterns of pain among subgroups of fibromyalgia patients. *British Journal of Medical Psychology* 71 (Pt. 2):185-194.

Laser T. (1998). [Comment on W. Hausotter: Fibromyalgia—a dispensable disease concept? (letter)] Zu W. Hausotter: Fibromyalgie—ein entbehrlicher krankheitsbegriff? *Versicherungsmedizin* 50(4):154-156.

Leonhardt T. (2000). [Fibromyalgia—a new name of an old "malady." Fatigue and pain syndrome with a historical background] Fibromyalgi—nytt namn pa gammal "sjuka". Trotthets-och smartsyndrom med historisk bakgrund. *Lakartidningen* 97(21):2618-2620, 2623-2624.

Leslie M. (1999). Fibromyalgia syndrome: A comprehensive approach to identification and management. *Clinical Excellence in Nurse Practice* 3(3):165-171.

Lilleaas UB. (1997). [Women's health—when the body breaks down (interview by Marianne Monsen)] Kvinnehelse—nar kroppen gar i stykker. *Tidsskr Sykepl* 85(20):42-43.

Lindberg NE; Lindberg E. (2000). [Use available knowledge—also when it is not complete. Current example: Chronic fatigue syndrome, fibromyalgia] Anvand befintlig kunskap—aven nar den ar ofullstandig aktuella exempel: Kroniskt trotthetssyndrom, fibromyalgi. *Lakartidningen* 97(21):2651-2652.

Littlejohn GO. (1996). Rheumatology. 2. Fibromyalgia syndrome. *Medical Journal of Australia* 7;165(7):387-391.

MacFarlane GJ; Croft PR; Schollum J; Silman AJ. (1996). Widespread pain: Is an improved classification possible? *Journal of Rheumatology* 23(9):1628-1632.

Maidannik VG. (1996). [The diagnosis and treatment of fibromyalgia] Diagnostika i lechenie fibromialgii. *Lik Sprava* (7-9):26-30.

Maier T. (1998). [Fibromyalgia (generalized tendomyopathy) in expert assessment] Die fibromyalgie (generalisierte tendomyopathie) in der begutachtungssituation. *Schweize Rundschrift Medizin Prax* 87(22):788-789.

Mailis A. (1996). Fibromyalgia 20 years later; what have we really accomplished? *Journal of Rheumatology* 23(1):193; discussion 193-194.

Makela MO. (1999). Is fibromyalgia a distinct clinical entity? The epidemiologist's evidence. *Baillieres Best Practice Research in Clinical Rheumatology* 13(3):415-419.

Mannerkorpi K; Kroksmark T; Ekdahl C. (1999). How patients with fibromyalgia experience their symptoms in everyday life. *Physiotherapy Research International* 4(2):110-122.

Marlowe SM. (1998). Calming the fire of fibromyalgia. *Advances in Nurse Practice* 6(1):51-53, 56.

Matsumoto Y. (1999). [Fibromyalgia syndrome]. *Nippon Rinsho* 57(2):364-369.

Maurizio SJ; Rogers JL. (1997). Recognizing and treating fibromyalgia. *Nurse Practice* 22(12):18-26, 28, 31; quiz 32-33.

Moldofsky H; Lue FA; Mously C; Roth-Schechter B; Reynolds WJ. (1996). The effect of zolpidem in patients with fibromyalgia: A dose ranging, double blind, placebo controlled, modified crossover study. *Journal of Rheumatology* 23(3):529-533.

Monroe BA. (1998). Fibromyalgia—a hidden link? *Journal of the American College of Nutrition* 17(3):300.

Neeck G. (1998). From the fibromyalgia challenge toward a new bio-psycho-social model of rheumatic diseases. *Zeitschrift Rheumatologie* 57 (Suppl. 2):A13-A16.

Neerinckx E; Van Houdenhove B; Lysen R; Vertommen H. (2000). What happens to the fibromyalgia concept? *Clinical Rheumatology* 19(1):1-5.

Nishikai M. (1999). [Fibromyalgia]. *Nippon Naika Gakkai Zasshi* 88(10):1937-1942.

Olin R; Lidbeck J. (1996). [Fibromyalgia—the explanatory mechanisms should be searched centrally, not peripherally (letter)] Fibromyalgi—forklaringarna skall sokas centralt, inte perifert. *Lakartidningen* 93(22):2125-2126.

Park JH; Phothimat P; Oates CT; Hernanz-Schulman M; Olsen NJ. (1998). Use of P-31 magnetic resonance spectroscopy to detect metabolic abnormalities in muscles of patients with fibromyalgia. *Arthritis and Rheumatism* 41(3):406-413.

Parziale JR; Chen JJ. (1996). Fibromyalgia. *Medical Health Rhode Island* 79(5):188-192.

Pasero CL. (1998). Understanding fibromyalgia syndrome. *American Journal of Nursing* 98(10):17-18.

Peloso PM. (1998). The fibromyalgia problem. *Journal of Rheumatology* 25(5):1024-1025; discussion 1028-1030.

Pocinki AG. (1997). Fireworks over fibromyalgia, CFS, and IBS. *Postgraduate Medicine* 102(6):43.

Pongratz DE; Sievers M. (2000). Fibromyalgia-symptom or diagnosis: A definition of the position. *Scandinavian Journal of Rheumatology* (Suppl. 113):3-7.

Potter PJ. (1997). Musculoskeletal complaints and fibromyalgia in patients attending a respiratory sleep disorders clinic. *Journal of Rheumatology* 24(8):1657-1658.

Proceedings of the International Fibromyalgia Conference (1998). Bad Nauheim, Germany, October 1997. *Zeitschrift Rheumatologie* 57 (Suppl. 2):V-X, 1-108.

Quintner JL; Cohen ML. (1997). Fibromyalgia syndrome. *Medical Journal of Australia* 166(3):168.

Quintner JL; Cohen ML. (1999). Fibromyalgia falls foul of a fallacy. *Lancet* 353(9158):1092-1094.

Rankin DB. (1999). The fibromyalgia syndrome: A consensus report. *New Zealand Medical Journal* 112(1080):18-19.

Raspe H. (1996). [Fibromyalgia—an artifact?] Fibromyalgie—ein artefakt? *Zeitschrift Rheumatologie* 55(1):1-3.

Raspe H; Croft P. (1995). Fibromyalgia. *Baillieres Clinical Rheumatology* 9(3):599-614.

Rau CL; Russell IJ. (2000). Is fibromyalgia a distinct clinical syndrome? *Current Reviews in Pain* 4(4):287-294.

Raymond MC; Brown JB. (2000). Experience of fibromyalgia. Qualitative study. *Canadian Family Physician* 46:1100-1106.

Reid GJ; Lang BA; McGrath PJ. (1997). Primary juvenile fibromyalgia: Psychological adjustment, family functioning, coping, and functional disability. *Arthritis and Rheumatism* 40(4):752-760.

Reiffenberger DH; Amundson LH. (1996). Fibromyalgia syndrome: A review. *American Family Physician* 53(5):1698-1712.

Reinhold-Keller E. (1997). [Diagnosis of fibromyalgia syndrome] Diagnose de fibromyalgiesyndroms. *Internist* (Berl) 38(10):993-994.

Rekola KE; Levoska S; Takala J; Keinanen-Kiukaanniemi S. (1997). Patients with neck and shoulder complaints and multisite musculoskeletal symptoms—a prospective study. *Journal of Rheumatology* 24(12):2424-2428.

Reveille JD. (1997). Soft-tissue rheumatism: Diagnosis and treatment. *American Journal of Medicine* 102(1A):23S-29S.

Reynolds WJ. (1996). Fibromyalgia 20 years later: What have we really accomplished? *Journal of Rheumatology* 23(1):192; discussion 193-194.

Robertson TJ. (1999). Misunderstood illnesses: Fibromyalgia and chronic fatigue syndrome. *Alta RN* 55(3):6-7.

Romano TJ. (1996). Fibromyalgia 20 years later: What have we really accomplished? *Journal of Rheumatology* 23(1):192; discussion 193-194.

Romano TJ. (1998). The fibromyalgia problem. *Journal of Rheumatology* 25(5):1026-1027; discussion 1028-1030.

Romano TJ. (1999). Patients with fibromyalgia must be treated fairly. *Archives of Internal Medicine* 159(20):2481-2483.

Russell IJ. (1999). Is fibromyalgia a distinct clinical entity? The clinical investigator's evidence. *Baillieres Best Practice Research in Clinical Rheumatology* 13(3):445-454.

Sabal N. (1997). Fireworks over fibromyalgia, CFS, and IBS. *Postgraduate Medicine* 102(6):44.

Safran S. (1998). Lack of control group deemed problematic in fibromyalgia pilot study. *Alternative Therapy Health Medicine* 4(5):114, 116.

Schaefer KM. (1997). Health patients of women with fibromyalgia. *Journal of Advanced Nursing* 26(3):565-571.

Scharf MB; Hauck M; Stover R; McDannold M; Berkowitz D. (1998). Effect of gamma-hydroxybutyrate on pain, fatigue, and the alpha sleep anomaly in patients with fibromyalgia. Preliminary report. *Journal of Rheumatology* 25(10):1986-1990.

Schuck JR; Chappell LT; Kindness G. (1997). Causal modeling and alternative medicine. *Alternative Therapy Health Medicine* 3(2):40-47.

Shelkovnikov IA; Krivoruchko BI. (1997). [Pathogenesis of fibromyalgia] Patogenez fibromialgii. *Patol Fiziol Eksp Ter* (1):41-42.

Shojania K. (2000). Rheumatology: 2. What laboratory tests are needed? *Canadian Medical Association Journal* 162(8):1157-1163.

Siegmeth W. (1999). [Panalgesia and the fibromyalgia concept] Panalgesie und das fibromyalgiekonzept. *Wien Medizin Wochenschrift* 149(19-20):558-560.

Simms RW. (1996). Fibromyalgia syndrome: Current concepts in pathophysiology, clinical features, and management. *Arthritis Care Research* 9(4):315-328.

Simms RW. (1998). Fibromyalgia is not a muscle disorder. *American Journal of Medical Sciences* 315(6):346-350.

Slavkin HC. (1997). Chronic disabling diseases and disorders: The challenges of fibromyalgia. *Journal of the American Dental Association* 128(11):1583-1589.

Smith MD. (1998). The fibromyalgia problem. *Journal of Rheumatology* 25(5):1027; discussion 1028-1030.

Smith WA. (1998). Fibromyalgia syndrome. *Nursing Clinics of North America* 33(4):653-669.

Solomon DH; Liang MH. (1997). Fibromyalgia: Scourge of humankind or bane of a rheumatologist's existence? *Arthritis and Rheumatism* 40(9):1553-1555.

Stoll AL. (2000). Fibromyalgia symptoms relieved by flupirtine: An open-label case series. *Psychosomatics* 41(4):371-372.

Tabeeva GR; Korotkova SB; Vein AM. (2000). [Fibromyalgia] Fibromialgiia. *Zh Nevrol Psikhiatr Im S S Korsakova* 100(4):69-77.

Thorson K. (1998). The fibromyalgia problem. *Journal of Rheumatology* 25(5):1023; discussion 1028-1030.

Thorson K. (1999). Is fibromyalgia a distinct clinical entity? The patient's evidence. *Baillieres Best Practice Research in Clinical Rheumatology* 13(3):463-467.

Turk DC; Okifuji A; Sinclair JD; Starz TW. (1996). Pain, disability, and physical functioning in subgroups of patients with fibromyalgia. *Journal of Rheumatology* 23(7):1255-1262.

Unger J. (1996). Fibromyalgia. *Journal of the American Academy of Nurse Practitioners* 8(1):27-29.

Unraveling a mysterious cause of pain. (1998). *Johns Hopkins Medical Letters on Health After 50* 10(4):3.

Uppgaard RO. (2000). Definition of myofascial face pain. *Journal of the American Dental Association* 131(7):854, 856, 858.

Van Santen-Hoeufft M. (1996). Typical fibromyalgia. *Clinical Rheumatology* 15(3):233-235.

Vree R. (1997). Fireworks over fibromyalgia, CFS, and IBS. *Postgraduate Medicine* 102(6):44.

Wallace DJ. (1997). The fibromyalgia syndrome. *Annals of Medicine* 29(1):9-21.

Wallace DJ. (1999). What constitutes a fibromyalgia expert? *Arthritis Care Research* 12(2):82-84.

Wallace DJ; Shapiro S; Panush RS. (1999). Update on fibromyalgia syndrome. *Bulletin of Rheumatic Diseases* 48(5):1-4.

Weber U. (1998). [Fibromyalgia (generalized tendomyopathy) expert assessment practice] Die fibromyalgie (generalisierte tendomyopathie) in der begutachtungssituation. *Schweize Rundschrift Medizin Prax* 87(24):856.

Wessely S; Hotopf M. (1999). Is fibromyalgia a distinct clinical entity? Historical and epidemiological evidence. *Baillieres Best Practice Research in Clinical Rheumatology* 13(3):427-436.

White KP; Harth M. (1998). The fibromyalgia problem. *Journal of Rheumatology* 25(5):1022-1023; discussion 1028-1030.

Wigley R. (1999). Can fibromyalgia be separated from regional pain syndrome affecting the arm? *Journal of Rheumatology* 26(3):515-516.

Wilke WS. (1996a). Fibromyalgia: More than a label. *Cleveland Clinic Journal of Medicine* 63(2):87-89.

Wilke WS. (1996b). Fibromyalgia. Recognizing and addressing the multiple interrelated factors. *Postgraduate Medicine* 100(1):153-156, 159, 163-166 passim.

Winfield JB. (1997). Fibromyalgia: What's next? *Arthritis Care Research* 10(4):219-221.

Wolfe F. (1997). The fibromyalgia problem. *Journal of Rheumatology* 24(7):1247-1249.

Wolfe F; Anderson J; Harkness D; Bennett RM; Caro XJ; Goldenberg DL; Russell IJ; Yunus MB. (1997). A prospective, longitudinal, multicenter study of service utilization and costs in fibromyalgia. *Arthritis and Rheumatism* 40(9):1560-1570.

Wootton JC. (2000). Fibromyalgia. *Journal of Women's Health and Gender Based Medicine* 9(5):571-573.

Xie X; Ye C. (1997). [Clinical analysis of 120 patients with fibromyalgia]. *Hunan I Ko Ta Hsueh Hsueh Pao* 22(2):167-170.

Zborovskii AB; Babaeva AR. (1998). [Diagnosis of primary fibromyalgia: Clinical criteria] Klinicheskie kriterii diagnoza pervichnoi fibromialgii. *Klin Med* (Mosk) 76(8):18-21.

*Fitness*

Natvig B; Bruusgaard D; Eriksen W. (1998). Physical leisure activity level and physical fitness among women with fibromyalgia. *Scandinavian Journal of Rheumatology* 27(5):337-341.

Nielens H; Boisset V; Masquelier E. (2000). Fitness and perceived exertion in patients with fibromyalgia syndrome. *Clinical Journal of Pain* 16(3):209-213.

Prevalence of leisure-time physical activity among persons with arthritis and other rheumatic conditions—United States, 1990-1991. (1997). *MMWR Morbidity and Mortality Weekly Report* 46(18):389-393.

## Functional Somatic Syndromes

Barsky AJ; Borus JF. (1999). Functional somatic syndromes. *Annals of Internal Medicine* 130(11):910-921.

Ford CV. (1997). Somatization and fashionable diagnoses: Illness as a way of life. *Scandinavian Journal of Work and Environmental Health* 23 (Suppl. 3):7-16.

Masi AT. (1998). Concepts of illness in populations as applied to fibromyalgia syndromes: A biopsychosocial perspective. *Zeitschrift Rheumatologie* 57 (Suppl. 2):31-35.

Robbins JM; Kirmayer LJ; Hemami S. (1997). Latent variable models of functional somatic distress. *Journal of Nervous and Mental Disorders* 185(10):606-615.

Walker EA; Katon WJ; Keegan D; Gardner G; Sullivan M. (1997). Predictors of physician frustration in the care of patients with rheumatological complaints. *General Hospital Psychiatry* 19(5):315-323.

## Gamma-hydroxybutyrate

Russell AS. (1999). Effect of gamma-hydroxybutyrate on pain, fatigue, and alpha sleep anomaly in patients with fibromyalgia. *Journal of Rheumatology* 26(12): 2712.

Scharf MB; Hauck M; Stover R; McDannold M; Berkowitz D. (1998). Effect of gamma-hydroxybutyrate on pain, fatigue, and the alpha sleep anomaly in patients with fibromyalgia. Preliminary report. *Journal of Rheumatology* 25(10): 1986-1990.

## Gender

Belilos E; Carsons S. (1998). Rheumatologic disorders in women. *Medicine Clinics of North America* 82(1):77-101.

Buckwalter JA; Lappin DR. (2000). The disproportionate impact of chronic arthralgia and arthritis among women. *Clinical Orthopedics* (372):159-168.

Burckhardt CS; Bjelle A. (1996). Perceived control: A comparison of women with fibromyalgia, rheumatoid arthritis, and systemic lupus erythematosus using a Swedish version of the Rheumatology Attitudes Index. *Scandinavian Journal of Rheumatology* 25(5):300-306.

Buskila D; Neumann L; Alhoashle A; Abu-Shakra M. (2000). Fibromyalgia syndrome in men. *Semin Arthritis and Rheumatism* 30(1):47-51.

Forseth KO; Forre O; Gran JT. (1999). A 5.5 year prospective study of self-reported musculoskeletal pain and of fibromyalgia in a female population: Significance and natural history. *Clinical Rheumatology* 18(2):114-121.

Forseth KO; Gran JT; Husby G. (1997). A population study of the incidence of fibromyalgia among women aged 26-55 yr. *British Journal of Rheumatology* 36(12):1318-1323.

Holtedahl R. (1999). [Spinal diseases and other musculoskeletal problems—too much of examination and treatment?] Rygglidelser og andre muskel-og skjelettlidelser—for mye utredning og behandling? *Tidsskr Nor Laegeforen* 119(20):3042.

Meisler JG. (1999). Chronic pain conditions in women. *Journal of Women's Health* 8(3):313-320.

Schaefer KM. (1997). Health patterns of women with fibromyalgia. *Journal of Advanced Nursing* 26(3):565-571.

Stormorken H; Brosstad F. (1999). [The "diffuse" health problems of women] Kvinners "ubestemte" helseplager. *Tidsskr Nor Laegeforen* 119(20):3043.

Yunus MB; Inanici F; Aldag JC; Mangold RF. (2000). Fibromyalgia in men: Comparison of clinical features with women. *Journal of Rheumatology* 27(2):485-490.

### Genetics

Ackenheil M. (1998). Genetics and pathophysiology of affective disorders: Relationship to fibromyalgia. *Zeitschrift Rheumatologie* 57 (Suppl. 2):5-7.

Buskila D. (2000). Fibromyalgia, chronic fatigue syndrome, and myofascial pain syndrome. *Current Opinions in Rheumatology* 12(2):113-123.

Buskila D; Neumann L. (1997). Fibromyalgia syndrome (FM) and nonarticular tenderness in relatives of patients with FM. *Journal of Rheumatology* 24(5):941-944.

Buskila D; Neumann L; Hazanov I; Carmi R. (1996). Familial aggregation in the fibromyalgia syndrome. *Seminars in Arthritis and Rheumatism* 26(3):605-611.

Klein R; Berg PA. (1995). High incidence of antibodies to 5-hydroxytryptamine, gangliosides and phospholipids in patients with chronic fatigue and fibromyalgia syndrome and their relatives: evidence for a clinical entity of both disorders. *European Journal of Medical Research* 1(1):21-26.

### Glucocorticoid

Ernberg M; Hedenberg-Magnusson B; Alstergren P; Kopp S. (1997). Short-term effect of glucocorticoid injection into the superficial masseter muscle of patients with chronic myalgia: A comparison between fibromyalgia and localized myalgia. *Journal of Orofacial Pain* 11(3):249-257.

### Growth Hormone

Bagge E; Bengtsson BA; Carlsson L; Carlsson J. (1998). Low growth hormone secretion in patients with fibromyalgia—a preliminary report on 10 patients and 10 controls. *Journal of Rheumatology* 25(1):145-148.

Bennett RM. (1998). Disordered growth hormone secretion in fibromyalgia: A review of recent findings and a hypothesized etiology. *Zeitschrift Rheumatologie* 57 (Suppl. 2):72-76.

Bennett RM; Clark SC; Walczyk J. (1998). A randomized, double-blind, placebo-controlled study of growth hormone in the treatment of fibromyalgia. *American Journal of Medicine* 104(3):227-231.

Berwaerts J; Moorkens G; Abs R. (1998). Secretion of growth hormone in patients with chronic fatigue syndrome. *Growth Hormone and IGF Research* 8 (Suppl. B): 127-129.

Dinser R; Halama T; Hoffmann A. (2000). Stringent endocrinological testing reveals subnormal growth hormone secretion in some patients with fibromyalgia syndrome but rarely severe growth hormone deficiency. *Journal of Rheumatology* 27(10):2482-2488.

Leal-Cerro A; Povedano J; Astorga R; Gonzalez M; Silva H; Garcia-Pesquera F; Casanueva FF; Dieguez C. (1999). The growth hormone (GH)-releasing hormone-GH-insulin-like growth factor-1 axis in patients with fibromyalgia syndrome. *Journal of Clinical Endocrinology and Metabolism* 84(9):3378-3381.

Schlienger JL; Goichot B. (1998). [Growth hormone: A magical potion?] Hormone de croissance: Potion magique? *Revue Medicine Interne* 19(4):279-285.

## *Gynecology*

Ostensen M; Schei B. (1997). Sociodemographic characteristics and gynecological disease in 40-42 year old women reporting musculoskeletal disease. *Scandinavian Journal of Rheumatology* 26(6):426-434.

ter Borg EJ; Gerards-Rociu E; Haanen HC; Westers P. (1999). High frequency of hysterectomies and appendectomies in fibromyalgia compared with rheumatoid arthritis: A pilot study. *Clinical Rheumatology* 18(1):1-3.

Wadsworth F; Kennedy S; Bradlow A; Barlow D; David J. (1995). Gynaecological symptoms in fibromyalgia. *British Journal of Rheumatology* 34(9):888-889.

## *Hair Electrolytes*

Ng SY. (1999). Hair calcium and magnesium levels in patients with fibromyalgia: A case center study. *Journal of Manipulative Physiology Therapy* 22(9):586-593.

## *Headache*

Bendtsen L. (2000). Central sensitization in tension-type headache—possible pathophysiological mechanisms. *Cephalalgia* 20(5):486-508.

Fox AW; Davis RL. (1998). Migraine chronobiology. *Headache* 38(6):436-441.

Nicolodi M; Sicuteri F. (1996). Fibromyalgia and migraine, two faces of the same mechanism. Serotonin as the common clue for pathogenesis and therapy. *Advances in Experimental Medical Biology* 398:373-379.

Nicolodi M; Volpe AR; Sicuteri F. (1998). Fibromyalgia and headache. Failure of serotonergic analgesia and N-methyl-D-aspartate-mediated neuronal plasticity: Their common clues. *Cephalalgia* 18 (Suppl. 21):41-44.

Okifuji A; Turk DC; Marcus DA. (1999). Comparison of generalized and localized hyperalgesia in patients with recurrent headache and fibromyalgia. *Psychosomatic Medicine* 61(6):771-780.

Paiva T; Batista A; Martins P; Martins A. (1995). The relationship between headaches and sleep disturbances. *Headache* 35(10):590-596.

Schepelmann K; Dannhausen M; Kotter I; Schabet M; Dichgans J. (1998). Exteroceptive suppression of temporalis muscle activity in patients with fibromyalgia, tension-type headache, and normal controls. *Electroencephalography and Clinical Neurophysiology* 107(3):196-199.

Stone RG; Wharton RB. (1997). Simultaneous multiple-modality therapy for tension headaches and neck pain. *Biomedical Instrumentation Technology* 31(3): 259-262.

### *Hearing*

Dohrenbusch R; Sodhi H; Lamprecht J; Genth E. (1997). Fibromyalgia as a disorder of perceptual organization? An analysis of acoustic stimulus processing in patients with widespread pain. *Zeitschrift Rheumatologie* 56(6):334-341.

Heller U; Becker EW; Zenner HP; Berg PA. (1998). [Incidence and clinical relevance of antibodies to phospholipids, serotonin and ganglioside in patients with sudden deafness and progressive inner ear hearing loss] Haufigkeit und klinische relevanz von antikorpern gegen phospholipide, serotonin und ganglioside bei patienten mit horsturz und progredienter innenohrschwerhorigkeit. *HNO* 46(6): 583-586.

Klein R; Berg PA. (1995). High incidence of antibodies to 5-hydroxytryptamine, gangliosides and phospholipids in patients with chronic fatigue and fibromyalgia syndrome and their relatives: Evidence for a clinical entity of both disorders. *European Journal of Medical Research* 1(1):21-26.

Kroner-Herwig B. (1997). [Fibromyalgia and the portals of perception] Fibromyalgie und die pforten der wahrnehmung. *Zeitschrift Rheumatologie* 56(6):319-321.

Rosenhall U; Johansson G; Orndahl G. (1996). Otoneurologic and audiologic findings in fibromyalgia. *Scandinavian Journal of Rehabilitative Medicine* 28(4): 225-232.

### *Hepatitis C*

Barkhuizen A; Bennett RM. (1997). Hepatitis C infection presenting with rheumatic manifestations. *Journal of Rheumatology* 24(6):1238-1239.

Buskila D. (2000). Hepatitis C-associated arthritis. *Current Opinions in Rheumatology* 12(4):295-299.

Buskila D; Shnaider A; Neumann L; Lorber M; Zilberman D; Hilzenrat N; Kuperman OJ; Sikuler E. (1998). Musculoskeletal manifestations and autoantibody profile in 90 hepatitis C virus infected Israeli patients. *Seminars in Arthritis and Rheumatism* 28(2):107-113.

Buskila D; Shnaider A; Neumann L; Zilberman D; Hilzenrat N; Sikuler E. (1997). Fibromyalgia in hepatitis C virus infection. Another infectious disease relationship. *Archives of Internal Medicine* 157(21):2497-2500.

Ferri C; Zignego AL. (2000). Relation between infection and autoimmunity in mixed cryoglobulinemia. *Current Opinions in Rheumatology* 12(1):53-60.

Jendro MC; Hulsemann JL; Zeidler H. (1997). [Hepatitis C virus in rheumatic diseases] Das Hepatitis C-virus und rheumatische erkrankungen. *Zeitschrift Rheumatologie* 56(5):276-286.

Killenberg PG. (2000). Extrahepatic manifestations of chronic hepatitis C. *Seminars in Gastrointestinal Diseases* 11(2):62-68.

Lovy MR; Starkebaum G; Uberoi S. (1996). Hepatitis C infection presenting with rheumatic manifestations: A mimic of rheumatoid arthritis. *Journal of Rheumatology* 23(6):979-983.

Rivera J; de Diego A; Trinchet M; Garcia Monforte A. (1997). Fibromyalgia-associated hepatitis C virus infection. *British Journal of Rheumatology* 36(9): 981-985.

## *Histocompatibility Linkage*

Yunus MB. (1998). Genetic factors in fibromyalgia syndrome. *Zeitschrift Rheumatologie* 57 (Suppl. 2):61-62.

Yunus MB; Khan MA; Rawlings KK; Green JR; Olson JM; Shah S. (1999). Genetic linkage analysis of multicase families with fibromyalgia syndrome. *Journal of Rheumatology* 26(2):408-412.

## *Homeopathy*

Jonas WB; Linde K; Ramirez G. (2000). Homeopathy and rheumatic disease. *Rheumatic Diseases Clinics of North America* 26(1):117-23, x.

## *Homocysteine*

Regland B; Andersson M; Abrahamsson L; Bagby J; Dyrehag LE; Gottfries CG. (1997). Increased concentrations of homocysteine in the cerebrospinal fluid in patients with fibromyalgia and chronic fatigue syndrome. *Scandinavian Journal of Rheumatology* 26(4):301-307.

### Hyaluronic Acid

Barkhuizen A; Bennett RM. (1999). Elevated levels of hyaluronic acid in the sera of women with fibromyalgia. *Journal of Rheumatology* 26(9):2063-2064.

Yaron I; Buskila D; Shirazi I; Neumann L; Elkayam O; Paran D; Yaron M. (1997). Elevated levels of hyaluronic acid in the sera of women with fibromyalgia. *Journal of Rheumatology* 24(11):2221-2224.

### Hydrocortisone

Teitelbaum JE; Bird B; Weiss A; Gould L. (1999). Low-dose hydrocortisone for chronic fatigue syndrome. *Journal of the American Medical Association* 281(20):1887-1888; discussion 1888-1889.

### Hyperkalemic Periodic Paralysis

Gotze FR; Thid S; Kyllerman M. (1998). Fibromyalgia in hyperkalemic periodic paralysis. *Scandinavian Journal of Rheumatology* 27(5):383-384.

### Hyperparathyroidism

Allerheiligen DA; Schoeber J; Houston RE; Mohl VK; Wildman KM. (1998). Hyperparathyroidism. *American Family Physician* 57(8):1795-1802, 1807-1808.

### Hypervigilance

Lorenz J. (1998). Hyperalgesia or hypervigilance? An evoked potential approach to the study of fibromyalgia syndrome. *Zeitschrift Rheumatologie* 57 (Suppl. 2): 19-22.

McDermid AJ; Rollman GB; McCain GA. (1996). Generalized hypervigilance in fibromyalgia: Evidence of perceptual amplification. *Pain* 66(2-3):133-144.

Peters ML; Vlaeyen JW; van Drunen C. (2000). Do fibromyalgia patients display hypervigilance for innocuous somatosensory stimuli? Application of a body scanning reaction time paradigm. *Pain* 86(3):283-292.

### Hypnosis

Wik G; Fischer H; Bragee B; Finer B; Fredrikson M. (1999). Functional anatomy of hypnotic analgesia: A PET study of patients with fibromyalgia. *European Journal of Pain* 3(1):7-12.

### Immunology

Bonaccorso S; Lin AH; Verkerk R; Van Hunsel F; Libbrecht I; Scharpe S; DeClerck L; Biondi M; Janca A; Maes M. (1998). Immune markers in fibromyalgia: Comparison with major depressed patients and normal volunteers. *Journal of Affective Disorders* 48(1):75-82.

Cole SW; Kemeny ME; Weitzman OB; Schoen M; Anton PA. (1999). Socially inhibited individuals show heightened DTH response during intense social engagement. *Brain, Behavior and Immunity* 13(2):187-200.

Maes M; Libbrecht I; Van Hunsel F; Lin AH; De Clerck L; Stevens W; Kenis G; de Jongh R; Bosmans E; Neels H. (1999). The immune-inflammatory pathophysiology of fibromyalgia: Increased serum soluble gp130, the common signal transducer protein of various neurotrophic cytokines. *Psychoneuroendocrinology* 24(4):371-383.

Samborski W; Lacki JK; Wiktorowicz KE. (1996). The lymphocyte phenotype in patients with primary fibromyalgia. *Upsala Journal of Medical Sciences* 101(3): 251-256.

Smart PA; Waylonis GW; Hackshaw KV. (1997). Immunologic profile of patients with fibromyalgia. *American Journal of Physical Medicine and Rehabilitation* 76(3):231-234.

### Inflammatory Bowel Disease

Buskila D; Odes LR; Neumann L; Odes HS. (1999). Fibromyalgia in inflammatory bowel disease. *Journal of Rheumatology* 26(5):1167-1171.

### Inflammatory Spinal Pain

Cantini F; Salvarani C; Olivieri I; Niccoli L; Padula A; Bellandi F; Palchetti R. (1998). Tuberculous spondylitis as a cause of inflammatory spinal pain: A report of 4 cases. *Clinical and Experimental Rheumatology* 16(3):305-308.

### Insulin-like Growth Factor-1

Bennett AL; Mayes DM; Fagioli LR; Guerriero R; Komaroff AL. (1997). Somatomedin C (insulin-like growth factor I) levels in patients with chronic fatigue syndrome. *Journal of Psychiatric Research* 31(1):91-96.

Buchwald D; Umali J; Stene M. (1996). Insulin-like growth factor-I (somatomedin C) levels in chronic fatigue syndrome and fibromyalgia. *Journal of Rheumatology* 23(4):739-742.

Dessein PH; Shipton EA; Joffe BI; Hadebe DP; Stanwix AE; Van der Merwe BA. (1999). Hyposecretion of adrenal androgens and the relation of serum adrenal steroids, serotonin and insulin-like growth factor-1 to clinical features in women with fibromyalgia. *Pain* 83(2):313-319.

Jacobsen S; Main K; Danneskiold-Samsoe B; Skakkebaek NE. (1995). A controlled study on serum insulin-like growth factor-I and urinary excretion of growth hormone in fibromyalgia. *Journal of Rheumatology* 22(6):1138-1140.

Leal-Cerro A; Povedano J; Astorga R; Gonzalez M; Silva H; Garcia-Pesquera F; Casanueva FF; Dieguez C. (1999). The growth hormone (GH)-releasing hormone-GH-insulin-like growth factor-1 axis in patients with fibromyalgia syndrome. *Journal of Clinical Endocrinology and Metabolism* 84(9):3378-3381.

Older SA; Battafarano DF; Danning CL; Ward JA; Grady EP; Derman S; Russell IJ. (1998). The effects of delta wave sleep interruption on pain thresholds and fibromyalgia-like symptoms in healthy subjects: Correlations with insulin-like growth factor I. *Journal of Rheumatology* 25(6):1180-1186.

Romano TJ. (1996). Controlled study on serum insulin-like growth factor I and urinary excretion of growth hormone in fibromyalgia. *Journal of Rheumatology* 23(1):194.

### *Interferon-alpha*

Russell IJ; Michalek JE; Kang YK; Richards AB. (1999). Reduction of morning stiffness and improvement in physical function in fibromyalgia syndrome patients treated sublingually with low doses of human interferon-alpha. *Journal of Interferon and Cytokine Research* 19(8):961-968.

Russell IJ; Vipraio GA; Michalek JE; Craig FE; Kang YK; Richards AB. (1999). Lymphocyte markers and natural killer cell activity in fibromyalgia syndrome: Effects of low-dose, sublingual use of human interferon-alpha. *Journal of Interferon and Cytokine Research* 19(8):969-978.

### *Interstitial Cystitis*

Alagiri M; Chottiner S; Ratner V; Slade D; Hanno PM. (1997). Interstitial cystitis: Unexplained associations with other chronic disease and pain syndromes. *Urology* 49(5A Suppl.):52-57.

Clauw DJ; Schmidt M; Radulovic D; Singer A; Katz P; Bresette J. (1997). The relationship between fibromyalgia and interstitial cystitis. *Journal of Psychiatric Research* 31(1):125-131.

### *Intramuscular Stimulation*

Chu J. (2000a). Early observations in radiculopathic pain control using electrodiagnostically derived new treatment techniques: Automated twitch-obtaining intramuscular stimulation (ATOIMS) and electrical twitch-obtaining intramuscular stimulation (ETOIMS). *Electromyography and Clinical Neurophysiology* 40(4):195-204.

Chu J. (2000b). The role of the monopolar electromyographic pin in myofascial pain therapy: automated twitch-obtaining intramuscular stimulation (ATOIMS) and electrical twitch-obtaining intramuscular stimulation (ETOIMS). *Electromyography and Clinical Neurophysiology* 39(8):503-511.

## Irritable Bowel Syndrome

Azpiroz F; Dapoigny M; Pace F; Muller-Lissner S; Coremans G; Whorwell P; Stockbrugger RW; Smout A. (2000). Nongastrointestinal disorders in the irritable bowel syndrome. *Digestion* 62(1):66-72.

Barton A; Pal B; Whorwell PJ; Marshall D. (1999). Increased prevalence of sicca complex and fibromyalgia in patients with irritable bowel syndrome. *American Journal of Gastroenterology* 94(7):1898-1901.

Chang L. (1998). The association of functional gastrointestinal disorders and fibromyalgia. *European Journal of Surgery* (Suppl. 583):32-36.

Chang L; Mayer EA; Johnson T; Fitzgerald LZ; Naliboff B. (2000). Differences in somatic perception in female patients with irritable bowel syndrome with and without fibromyalgia. *Pain* 84(2-3):297-307.

Chun A; Desautels S; Slivka A; Mitrani C; Starz T; DiLorenzo C; Wald A. (1999). Visceral algesia in irritable bowel syndrome, fibromyalgia, and sphincter of oddi dysfunction, type III. *Digestive Disease Sciences* 44(3):631-636.

Mayer EA; Fass R; Fullerton S. (1998). Intestinal and extraintestinal symptoms in functional gastrointestinal disorders. *European Journal of Surgery* (Suppl. 583): 29-31.

Sivri A; Cindas A; Dincer F; Sivri B. (1996). Bowel dysfunction and irritable bowel syndrome in fibromyalgia patients. *Clinical Rheumatology* 15(3):283-286.

Sperber AD; Atzmon Y; Neumann L; Weisberg I; Shalit Y; Abu-Shakrah M; Fich A; Buskila D. (1999). Fibromyalgia in the irritable bowel syndrome: Studies of prevalence and clinical implications. *American Journal of Gastroenterology* 94(12):3541-3546.

Sperber AD; Carmel S; Atzmon Y; Weisberg I; Shalit Y; Neumann L; Fich A; Buskila D. (1999). The sense of coherence index and the irritable bowel syndrome. A cross-sectional comparison among irritable bowel syndrome patients with and without coexisting fibromyalgia, irritable bowel syndrome non-patients, and controls. *Scandinavian Journal of Gastroenterology* 34(3):259-263.

Sperber AD; Carmel S; Atzmon Y; Weisberg I; Shalit Y; Neumann L; Fich A; Friger M; Buskila D. (2000). Use of the Functional Bowel Disorder Severity Index (FBDSI) in a study of patients with the irritable bowel syndrome and fibromyalgia. *American Journal of Gastroenterology* 95(4):995-998.

## Joint Hypermobility

Acasuso-Diaz M; Collantes-Estevez E. (1998). Joint hypermobility in patients with fibromyalgia syndrome. *Arthritis Care Research* 11(1):39-42.

Fitzcharles MA. (2000). Is hypermobility a factor in fibromyalgia? *Journal of Rheumatology* 27(7):1587-1589.

Hudson N; Fitzcharles MA; Cohen M; Starr MR; Esdaile JM. (1998). The association of soft-tissue rheumatism and hypermobility. *British Journal of Rheumatology* 37(4):382-386.

Hudson N; Starr MR; Esdaile JM; Fitzcharles MA. (1995). Diagnostic associations with hypermobility in rheumatology patients. *British Journal of Rheumatology* 34(12):1157-1161.

Karaaslan Y; Haznedaroglu S; Ozturk M. (2000). Joint hypermobility and primary fibromyalgia: A clinical enigma. *Journal of Rheumatology* 27(7):1774-1776.

Klemp P. (1997). Hypermobility. *Annals of Rheumatic Diseases* 56(10):573-575.

Lai S; Goldman JA; Child AH; Engel A; Lamm SH. (2000). Fibromyalgia, hypermobility, and breast implants. *Journal of Rheumatology* 27(9):2237-2241.

## *Juvenile Fibromyalgia*

Breau LM; McGrath PJ; Ju LH. (1999). Review of juvenile primary fibromyalgia and chronic fatigue syndrome. *Journal of Developmental Behavioral Pediatrics* 20(4):278-288.

Buskila D. (1996). Fibromyalgia in children—lessons from assessing nonarticular tenderness. *Journal of Rheumatology* 23(12):2017-2079.

Cassidy JT. (1998). Progress in diagnosis and understanding chronic pain syndromes in children and adolescents. *Adolescent Medicine* 9(1):101-114, vi.

Clark P; Burgos-Vargas R; Medina-Palma C; Lavielle P; Marina FF. (1998). Prevalence of fibromyalgia in children: A clinical study of Mexican children. *Journal of Rheumatology* 25(10):2009-2014.

Gedalia A; Garcia CO; Molina JF; Bradford NJ; Espinoza LR. (2000). Fibromyalgia syndrome: Experience in a pediatric rheumatology clinic. *Clinical and Experimental Rheumatology* 18(3):415-419.

Haavet OR; Grunfeld B. (1997). [Are life experiences of children significant for the development of somatic disease? A literature review] Er barns livserfaringer av betydning for somatisk sykdomsutvikling? En litteraturoversikt. *Tidsskr Nor Laegeforen* 117(25):3644-3647.

Kujala UM; Taimela S; Viljanen T. (1999). Leisure physical activity and various pain symptoms among adolescents. *British Journal of Sports Medicine* 33(5): 325-328.

Kulig JW. (1991). Chronic fatigue syndrome and fibromyalgia in adolescence. *Adolescent Medicine* 2(3):473-484.

Mikkelsson M. (1999). One year outcome of preadolescents with fibromyalgia. *Journal of Rheumatology* 26(3):674-682.

Mikkelsson M; Salminen JJ; Kautiainen H. (1997). Non-specific musculoskeletal pain in preadolescents. Prevalence and 1-year persistence. *Pain* 73(1):29-35.

Mikkelsson M; Sourander A; Piha J; Salminen JJ. (1997). Psychiatric symptoms in preadolescents with musculoskeletal pain and fibromyalgia. *Pediatrics* 100(2 Pt. 1):220-227.

Reid GJ; Lang BA; McGrath PJ. (1997). Primary juvenile fibromyalgia: Psychological adjustment, family functioning, coping, and functional disability. *Arthritis and Rheumatism* 40(4):752-760.

Roizenblatt S; Tufik S; Goldenberg J; Pinto LR; Hilario MO; Feldman D. (1997). Juvenile fibromyalgia: Clinical and polysomnographic aspects. *Journal of Rheumatology* 24(3):579-585.

Rusy LM; Harvey SA; Beste DJ. (1999). Pediatric fibromyalgia and dizziness: Evaluation of vestibular function. *Journal of Developmental Behavioral Pediatrics* 20(4):211-215.

Schanberg LE; Keefe FJ; Lefebvre JC; Kredich DW; Gil KM. (1996). Pain coping strategies in children with juvenile primary fibromyalgia syndrome: Correlation with pain, physical function, and psychological distress. *Arthritis Care Research* 9(2):89-96.

Schanberg LE; Keefe FJ; Lefebvre JC; Kredich DW; Gil KM. (1998). Social context of pain in children with Juvenile primary fibromyalgia syndrome: Parental pain history and family environment. *Clinical Journal of Pain* 14(2):107-115.

Schikler KN. (2000). Is it juvenile rheumatoid arthritis or fibromyalgia? *Medicine Clinics of North America* 84(4):967-982.

Sherry DD. (1997). Musculoskeletal pain in children. *Current Opinions in Rheumatology* 9(5):465-470.

Sieb JP; Dorfler P; Tolksdorf K; Jakschik J. (1997). Endplate ultrastructure in a case of primary fibromyalgia. *Clinical Rheumatology* 16(6):637-638.

Siegel DM; Janeway D; Baum J. (1998). Fibromyalgia syndrome in children and adolescents: Clinical features at presentation and status at follow-up. *Pediatrics* 101(3 Pt. 1):377-382.

Tayag-Kier CE; Keenan GF; Scalzi LV; Schultz B; Elliott J; Zhao RH; Arens R. (2000). Sleep and periodic limb movement in sleep in juvenile fibromyalgia. *Pediatrics* 106(5):E70.

*Keratoconjunctivitis Sicca*

Barton A; Pal B; Whorwell PJ; Marshall D. (1999). Increased prevalence of sicca complex and fibromyalgia in patients with irritable bowel syndrome. *American Journal of Gastroenterology* 94(7):1898-1901.

Gunaydin I; Terhorst T; Eckstein A; Daikeler T; Kanz L; Kotter I. (1999). Assessment of keratoconjunctivitis sicca in patients with fibromyalgia: Results of a prospective study. *Rheumatology International* 19(1-2):7-9.

*Ketamine*

Graven-Nielsen T; Aspegren Kendall S; Henriksson KG; Bengtsson M; Sorensen J; Johnson A; Gerdle B; Arendt-Nielsen L. (2000). Ketamine reduces muscle pain, temporal summation, and referred pain in fibromyalgia patients. *Pain* 85(3):483-491.

Oye I; Rabben T; Fagerlund TH. (1996). [Analgesic effect of ketamine in a patient with neuropathic pain] Analgetisk effekt av ketamin hos en pasient med neuropatiske smerter. *Tidsskr Nor Laegeforen* 116(26):3130-3131.

## Klebsiella

Toivanen P; Hansen DS; Mestre F; Lehtonen L; Vaahtovuo J; Vehma M; Mottonen T; Saario R; Luukkainen R; Nissila M. (1999). Somatic serogroups, capsular types, and species of fecal Klebsiella in patients with ankylosing spondylitis. *Journal of Clinical Microbiology* 37(9):2808-2812.

## *Laser Therapy*

Longo L; Simunovic Z; Postiglione M; Postiglione M. (1997). Laser therapy for fibromyositic rheumatisms. *Journal of Clinical Laser Medicine Surgery* 15(5):217-220.

## *Leiomyosarcoma*

De Tomas Palacios J; Sanchez Sabate E; Turegano Fuentes F; Zabay JM. (1995). [Retroperitoneal leiomyosarcoma in a patient with fibromyalgia] Leiomio-sarcoma retroperitoneal en una paciente con fibromialgia. *Anales de Medicina Interna* 12(12):617-618.

## *Lidocaine*

Figuerola ML; Loe W; Sormani M; Barontini M. (1998). Met-enkephalin increase in patients with fibromyalgia under local treatment. *Functional Neurology* 13(4):291-295.

Koppert W; Zeck S; Sittl R; Likar R; Knoll R; Schmelz M. (1998). Low-dose lidocaine suppresses experimentally induced hyperalgesia in humans. *Anesthesiology* 89(6):1345-1353.

Scudds RA; Janzen V; Delaney G; Heck C; McCain GA; Russell AL; Teasell RW; Varkey G; Woodbury MG. (1995). The use of topical 4 percent lidocaine in spheno-palatine ganglion blocks for the treatment of chronic muscle pain syndromes: a randomized, controlled trial. *Pain* 62(1):69-77.

## *Light Treatment*

Pearl SJ; Lue F; MacLean AW; Heslegrave RJ; Reynolds WJ; Moldofsky H. (1996). The effects of bright light treatment on the symptoms of fibromyalgia. *Journal of Rheumatology* 23(5):896-902.

Tabeeva GR; Levin IAI; Korotkova SB; Khanunov IG. (1998). [Treatment of fibromyalgia] Lechenie fibromialgii. *Zh Nevrol Psikhiatr Im S S Korsakova* 98(4):40-43.

## Magnesium

Eisinger J; Zakarian H; Pouly E; Plantamura A; Ayavou T. (1996). Protein peroxidation, magnesium deficiency and fibromyalgia. *Magnesium Research* 9(4):313-316.

Moorkens G; Manuel y Keenoy B; Vertommen J; Meludu S; Noe M; De Leeuw I. (1997). Magnesium deficit in a sample of the Belgian population presenting with chronic fatigue. *Magnesium Research* 10(4):329-337.

## Massage

Brattberg G. (1999). Connective tissue massage in the treatment of fibromyalgia. *European Journal of Pain* 3(3):235-244.

## Masticatory Myofascial Pain

Cimino R; Michelotti A; Stradi R; Farinaro C. (1998). Comparison of clinical and psychologic features of fibromyalgia and masticatory myofascial pain. *Journal of Orofacial Pain* 12(1):35-41.

## Medicinal Baths

Ammer K; Melnizky P. (1999). [Medicinal baths for treatment of generalized fibromyalgia] Medizinalbader zur therapie der generalisierten fibromyalgie. *Forschrift Komplementarmedizin* 6(2):80-85.

## Melatonin

Citera G; Arias MA; Maldonado-Cocco JA; Lazaro MA; Rosemffet MG; Brusco LI; Scheines EJ; Cardinalli DP. (2000). The effect of melatonin in patients with fibromyalgia: A pilot study. *Clinical Rheumatology* 19(1):9-13.

Korszun A; Sackett-Lundeen L; Papadopoulos E; Brucksch C; Masterson L; Engelberg NC; Haus E; Demitrack MA; Crofford L. (1999). Melatonin levels in women with fibromyalgia and chronic fatigue syndrome. *Journal of Rheumatology* 26(12):2675-2680.

Press J; Phillip M; Neumann L; Barak R; Segev Y; Abu-Shakra M; Buskila D. (1998). Normal melatonin levels in patients with fibromyalgia syndrome. *Journal of Rheumatology* 25(3):551-555.

Webb SM. (1998). Fibromyalgia and melatonin: Are they related? *Clinical Endocrinology* (Oxford) 49(2):161-162.

Wikner J; Hirsch U; Wetterberg L; Rojdmark S. (1998). Fibromyalgia—a syndrome associated with decreased nocturnal melatonin secretion. *Clinical Endocrinology* (Oxford) 49(2):179-183.

## Mitochondrial Myopathy

Benito-Leon J; Berbel A; Porta-Estessam J; Martinez A; Arenas J. (1996). [Fibromyalgia in right half of the body as the onset of mitochondrial cytopathy. Letter] Fibromialgia en hemicuerpo derecho como forma de presentacion de una citopatia mitocondrial. *Revista Neurologica* 24(134):1303-1304.

Villanova M; Selvi E; Malandrini A; Casali C; Santorelli FM; De Stefano R; Marcolongo R. (1999). Mitochondrial myopathy mimicking fibromyalgia syndrome. *Muscle Nerve* 22(2):289-291.

## Moclobemide

Hannonen P; Malminiemi K; Yli-Kerttula U; Isomeri R; Roponen P. (1998). A randomized, double-blind, placebo-controlled study of moclobemide and amitriptyline in the treatment of fibromyalgia in females without psychiatric disorder. *British Journal of Rheumatology* 37(12):1279-1286.

## Motor Cortical Dysfunction

Burgunder JM. (1998). Pathophysiology of akinetic movement disorders: A paradigm for studies in fibromyalgia? *Zeitschrift Rheumatologie* 57 (Suppl. 2):27-30.

Ivanichev GA; Starosel'tseva NG. (2000). [Fibromyalgia (generalized tendomyopathy): Defect of a program of movements and their realization] Fibromialgiia (generalizovannaia tendomiopatiia)—defekt programmy postroeniia i ispolneniia dvizheniia. *Zh Nevrol Psikhiatr Im S S Korsakova* 100(4):54-61.

Salerno A; Thomas E; Olive P; Blotman F; Picot MC; Georgesco M. (2000). Motor cortical dysfunction disclosed by single and double magnetic stimulation in patients with fibromyalgia. *Clinical Neurophysiology* 111(6):994-1001.

## Mud Packs

Bellometti S; Galzigna L. (1999). Function of the hypothalamic adrenal axis in patients with fibromyalgia syndrome undergoing mud-pack treatment. *International Journal of Clinical Pharmacology Research* 19(1):27-33.

## Muscle Abnormalities

Argov Z; Lofberg M; Arnold DL. (2000). Insights into muscle diseases gained by phosphorus magnetic resonance spectroscopy. *Muscle Nerve* 23(9):1316-1334.

Borman P; Celiker R; Hascelik Z. (1999). Muscle performance in fibromyalgia syndrome. *Rheumatology International* 19(1-2):27-30.

Graven-Nielsen T; Svensson P; Arendt-Nielsen L. (1997). Effects of experimental muscle pain on muscle activity and co-ordination during static and dynamic motor function. *Electroencephalography and Clinical Neurophysiology* 105(2): 156-164.

Hakkinen A; Hakkinen K; Hannonen P; Alen M. (2000). Force production capacity and acute neuromuscular responses to fatiguing loading in women with fibromyalgia are not different from those of healthy women. *Journal of Rheumatology* 27(5):1277-1282.

Henriksson KG; Backman E; Henriksson C; de Laval JH. (1996). Chronic regional muscular pain in women with precise manipulation work. A study of pain characteristics, muscle function, and impact on daily activities. *Scandinavian Journal of Rheumatology* 25(4):213-223.

Jacobsen S. (1998). Physical biodynamics and performance capacities of muscle in patients with fibromyalgia syndrome. *Zeitschrift Rheumatologie* 57 (Suppl. 2): 43-46.

Norregaard J. (1998). Muscle function, psychometric scoring and prognosis in patients with widespread pain and tenderness (fibromyalgia). *Danish Medical Bulletin* 45(3):256-267.

Norregaard J; Bulow PM; Vestergaard-Poulsen P; Thomsen C; Danneskiold-Samoe B. (1995). Muscle strength, voluntary activation and cross-sectional muscle area in patients with fibromyalgia. *British Journal of Rheumatology* 34(10):925-931.

Olsen NJ; Park JH. (1998). Skeletal muscle abnormalities in patients with fibromyalgia. *American Journal of Medical Sciences* 315(6):351-358.

Park JH; Phothimat P; Oates CT; Hernanz-Schulman M; Olsen NJ. (1998). Use of P-31 magnetic resonance spectroscopy to detect metabolic abnormalities in muscles of patients with fibromyalgia. *Arthritis and Rheumatism* 41(3):406-413.

Pongratz DE; Spath M. (1998). Morphologic aspects of fibromyalgia. *Zeitschrift Rheumatologie* 57 Suppl 2:47-51.

Sann H; Pierau FK. (1998). Efferent functions of C-fiber nociceptors. *Zeitschrift Rheumatologie* 57 (Suppl. 2):8-13.

Simms RW. (1996). Is there muscle pathology in fibromyalgia syndrome? *Rheumatic Diseases Clinics of North America* 22(2):245-266.

Sprott H; Rzanny R; Reichenbach JR; Kaiser WA; Hein G; Stein G. (2000). 31P magnetic resonance spectroscopy in fibromyalgic muscle. *Rheumatology* (Oxford) 39(10):1121-1125.

Strobel ES; Krapf M; Suckfull M; Bruckle W; Fleckenstein W; Muller W. (1997). Tissue oxygen measurement and 31P magnetic resonance spectroscopy in patients with muscle tension and fibromyalgia. *Rheumatology International* 16(5):175-180.

Thorsteinsdottir B; Rafnsdottir S; Geirsson AJ; Sigurjonsson SV; Kjeld M. (1998). No difference in ubiquinone concentration of muscles and blood in fibromyalgia patients and healthy controls. *Clinical and Experimental Rheumatology* 16(4):513-514.

Vestergaard-Poulsen P; Thomsen C; Norregaard J; Bulow P; Sinkjaer T; Henriksen O. (1995). 31P NMR spectroscopy and electromyography during exercise and recovery in patients with fibromyalgia. *Journal of Rheumatology* 22(8):1544-1551.

Wachter KC; Kaeser HE; Guhring H; Ettlin TM; Mennet P; Muller W. (1996). Muscle damping measured with a modified pendulum test in patients with fibromyalgia, lumbago, and cervical syndrome. *Spine* 21(18):2137-2142.

## *Mycoplasma*

Choppa PC; Vojdani A; Tagle C; Andrin R; Magtoto L. (1998). Multiplex PCR for the detection of *Mycoplasma fermentans, M. hominis* and *M. penetrans* in cell cultures and blood samples of patients with chronic fatigue syndrome. *Molecular and Cellular Probes* 12(5):301-308.

Nasralla M; Haier J; Nicolson GL. (1999). Multiple mycoplasmal infections detected in blood of patients with chronic fatigue syndrome and/or fibromyalgia syndrome. *European Journal of Clinical Microbiology and Infectious Diseases* 18(12):859-865.

## *Myoadenylate Deaminase Deficiency*

Marin R; Connick E. (1997). Tension myalgia versus myoadenylate deaminase deficiency: A case report. *Archives of Physical Medicine Rehabilitation* 78(1): 95-97.

## *Myofascial Pain Syndrome*

Aronoff GM. (1998). Myofascial pain syndrome and fibromyalgia: A critical assessment and alternate view. *Clinical Journal of Pain* 14(1):74-85.

Bernstein WJ. (1997). Myofascial pain and fibromyalgia syndromes. *Neurology* 48(6):1738; discussion 1741-1742.

Bohr T. (1996). Problems with myofascial pain syndrome and fibromyalgia syndrome. *Neurology* 46(3):593-597.

Cimino R; Michelotti A; Stradi R; Farinaro C. (1998). Comparison of clinical and psychologic features of fibromyalgia and masticatory myofascial pain. *Journal of Orofacial Pain* 12(1):35-41.

Dao TT; Reynolds WJ; Tenenbaum HC. (1997). Comorbidity between myofascial pain of the masticatory muscles and fibromyalgia. *Journal of Orofacial Pain* 11(3):232-241.

Dao T; Reynolds WJ; Tenenbaum HC. (1998). Comorbidity between myofascial pain of the masticatory muscles and fibromyalgia. *Alpha Omegan* 91(2):29-37.

Fishbain DA; Rosomoff HL. (1996). Myofascial pain syndrome and post-traumatic fibromyalgia: Comment on the article by Wolfe. *Arthritis Care Research* 9(2): 157-158.

Galer BS. (1997). Myofascial pain and fibromyalgia syndrome. *Neurology* 48(6): 1739; discussion 1741-1742.

Gantz NM; Fukuda K. (1997). Myofascial pain and fibromyalgia syndrome. *Neurology* 48(6):1738-1739; discussion 1741-1742.

Goldenberg DL. (1996). Fibromyalgia, chronic fatigue syndrome, and myofascial pain. *Current Opinions in Rheumatology* 8(2):113-123.

Harden RN; Bruehl SP; Gass S; Niemiec C; Barbick B. (2000). Signs and symptoms of the myofascial pain syndrome: a national survey of pain management providers. *Clinical Journal of Pain* 16(1):64-72.

Long DM Jr. (1997). Myofascial pain and fibromyalgia syndrome. *Neurology* 48(6):1740-1741; discussion 1741-1742.

Nye DA. (1997). Myofascial pain and fibromyalgia syndrome. *Neurology* 48(6): 1739; discussion 1741-1742.

Perle SM. (1996). Tender points/fibromyalgia vs. trigger points/myofascial pain syndrome: A need for clarity in terminology and differential diagnosis. *Journal of Manipulative Physiology Therapy* 19(2):146-147.

Pongratz DE; Spath M. (1998). [Myofascial pain syndrome—frequent occurrence and often misdiagnosed] Das myofasziale schmerzsyndrom—haufig vorhanden und haufig verkannt. *Fortschrift Medizin* 116(27):24-29.

Raphael KG; Marbach JJ. (2000). Comorbid fibromyalgia accounts for reduced fecundity in women with myofascial face pain. *Clinical Journal of Pain* 16(1): 29-36.

Raphael KG; Marbach JJ; Klausner J. (2000). Myofascial face pain. Clinical characteristics of those with regional vs. widespread pain. *Journal of the American Dental Association* 131(2):161-171.

Romano TJ. (1997). Myofascial pain and fibromyalgia syndrome. *Neurology* 48(6): 1739-1740; discussion 1741-1742.

Schneider MJ. (1995). Tender points/fibromyalgia vs. trigger points/myofascial pain syndrome: A need for clarity in terminology and differential diagnosis. *Journal of Manipulative Physiology Therapy* 18(6):398-406.

### Natural Killer Cells

Barker E; Fujimura SF; Fadem MB; Landay AL; Levy JA. (1994). Immunologic abnormalities associated with chronic fatigue syndrome. *Clinical Infectious Diseases* 18(Suppl. 1):S136-S141.

DuBois E. (1986). Gamma globulin therapy for chronic mononucleosis syndrome. *AIDS Research and Human Retroviruses* 2(1):S191-S195.

Gupta S; Vayuvegula B. (1991). A comprehensive immunological analysis in chronic fatigue syndrome. *Scandinavian Journal of Immunology* 33(3):319-327.

Kibler R; Lucas DO; Hicks MJ; Poulos BT; Jones JF. (1985). Immune function in chronic active Epstein-Barr virus infection. *Journal of Clinical Immunology* 5:46-54.

Klimas N; Salvato F; Morgan R; Fletcher MA. (1990). Immunologic abnormalities in chronic fatigue syndrome. *Journal of Clinical Microbiology* 28(6):1403-1410.

Lekander M; Fredrikson M; Wik G. (2000). Neuroimmune relations in patients with fibromyalgia: A positron emission tomography study. *Neurosciences Letters* 282(3):193-196.

Morrison LJ; Behan WH; Behan PO. (1991). Changes in natural killer cell phenotype in patients with post-viral fatigue syndrome. *Clinical and Experimental Immunology* 83:441-446.

Ojo-Amaise EA; Conley EJ; Peters JB. (1994). Decreased natural killer cell activity is associated with severity of chronic fatigue immune deficiency syndrome. *Clinical Infectious Diseases* 18:S157-S159.

Patarca R; Fletcher MA; Podack ER. (1995). Cytolytic cell functions. In *Manual of Clinical Laboratory Immunology*. Rose NR, de Macario EC, Folds JD, Lane HC, Nakamura RM (eds.), Washington DC, American Society for Microbiology, pp. 296-303.

Russell IJ; Vipraio GA; Michalek JE; Craig FE; Kang YK; Richards AB. (1999). Lymphocyte markers and natural killer cell activity in fibromyalgia syndrome: Effects of low-dose, sublingual use of human interferon-alpha. *Journal of Interferon and Cytokine Research* 19(8):969-978.

See DM; Broumand N; Sahl L; Tilles JG. (1997). In vitro effect of echinacea and ginseng on natural killer and antibody-dependent cell cytotoxicity in healthy subjects and chronic fatigue syndrome or acquired immunodeficiency syndrome. *Immunopharmacology* 35:229-235.

Straus SE; Tosato G; Armstrong G; Lawley T; Preble OT; Henle W; Davey R; Pearson G; Epstein J; Brus I. (1985). Persisting illness and fatigue in adults with evidence of Epstein-Barr virus infection. *Annals of Internal Medicine* 102:7-16.

Whiteside TL; Friberg D. (1998). Natural killer cells and natural killer cell activity in chronic fatigue syndrome. *American Journal of Medicine* 1998; 105(3A): 27S-34S.

*Neck Support*

Ambrogio N; Cuttiford J; Lineker S; Li L. (1998). A comparison of three types of neck support in fibromyalgia patients. *Arthritis Care Research* 11(5):405-410.

*Nerve Growth Factor*

Giovengo SL; Russell IJ; Larson AA. (1999). Increased concentrations of nerve growth factor in cerebrospinal fluid of patients with fibromyalgia. *Journal of Rheumatology* 26(7):1564-1569.

*Neuroendocrinology*

Adler GK; Kinsley BT; Hurwitz S; Mossey CJ; Goldenberg DL. (1999). Reduced hypothalamic-pituitary and sympathoadrenal responses to hypoglycemia in women with fibromyalgia syndrome. *American Journal of Medicine* 106(5): 534-543.

Akkus S; Delibas N; Tamer MN. (2000). Do sex hormones play a role in fibromyalgia? *Rheumatology* (Oxford) 39(10):1161-1163.

Anderberg UM. (2000). Comment on: Johns and Littlejohn, The role of sex hormones in pain response. *Pain* 87(1):109-111.

Anisman H; Baines MG; Berczi I; Bernstein CN; Blennerhassett MG; Gorczynski RM; Greenberg AH; Kisil FT; Mathison RD; Nagy E; Nance DM; Perdue MH; Pomerantz DK; Sabbadini ER; Stanisz A; Warrington RJ. (1996). Neuroimmune mechanisms in health and disease: 2. Disease. *Canadian Medical Association Journal* 155(8):1075-1082.

Bellometti S; Galzigna L. (1999). Function of the hypothalamic adrenal axis in patients with fibromyalgia syndrome undergoing mud-pack treatment. *International Journal of Clinical Pharmacology Research* 19(1):27-33.

Bennett RM; Cook DM; Clark SR; Burckhardt CS; Campbell SM. (1997). Hypothalamic-pituitary-insulin-like growth factor-I axis dysfunction in patients with fibromyalgia. *Journal of Rheumatology* 24(7):1384-1389.

Bradley LA; McKendree-Smith NL; Alarcon GS. (2000). Pain complaints in patients with fibromyalgia versus chronic fatigue syndrome. *Current Reviews on Pain* 4(2):148-157.

Clauw DJ; Chrousos GP. (1997). Chronic pain and fatigue syndromes: Overlapping clinical and neuroendocrine features and potential pathogenic mechanisms. *Neuroimmunomodulation* 4(3):134-153.

Crofford LJ. (1998a). The hypothalamic-pituitary-adrenal stress axis in fibromyalgia and chronic fatigue syndrome. *Zeitschrift Rheumatologie* 57 (Suppl. 2):67-71.

Crofford LJ. (1998b). Neuroendocrine abnormalities in fibromyalgia and related disorders. *American Journal of Medical Sciences* 315(6):359-366.

Crofford LJ; Demitrack MA. (1996). Evidence that abnormalities of central neurohormonal systems are key to understanding fibromyalgia and chronic fatigue syndrome. *Rheumatic Diseases Clinics of North America* 22(2):267-284.

Crofford LJ; Engleberg NC; Demitrack MA. (1996). Neurohormonal perturbations in fibromyalgia. *Baillieres Clinical Rheumatology* 10(2):365-378.

Demitrack MA. (1997). Neuroendocrine correlates of chronic fatigue syndrome: A brief review. *Journal of Psychiatric Research* 31(1):69-82.

Demitrack MA; Crofford LJ. (1998). Evidence for and pathophysiologic implications of hypothalamic-pituitary-adrenal axis dysregulation in fibromyalgia and chronic fatigue syndrome. *Annals of the New York Academy of Sciences* 840: 684-697.

Dessein PH; Shipton EA; Stanwix AE; Joffe BI. (2000). Neuroendocrine deficiency-mediated development and persistence of pain in fibromyalgia: A promising paradigm? *Pain* 86(3):213-215.

Griep EN; Boersma JW; Lentjes EG; Prins AP; van der Korst JK; de Kloet ER. (1998). Function of the hypothalamic-pituitary-adrenal axis in patients with fibromyalgia and low back pain. *Journal of Rheumatology* 25(7):1374-1381.

Hapidou EG; Rollman GB. (1998). Menstrual cycle modulation of tender points. *Pain* 77(2):151-161.

Heim C; Ehlert U; Hellhammer DH. (2000). The potential role of hypocortisolism in the pathophysiology of stress-related bodily disorders. *Psychoneuroendocrinology* 25(1):1-35.

Korszun A; Young EA; Engleberg NC; Masterson L; Dawson EC; Spindler K; McClure LA; Brown MB; Crofford LJ. (2000). Follicular phase hypothalamic-pituitary-gonadal axis function in women with fibromyalgia and chronic fatigue syndrome. *Journal of Rheumatology* 27(6):1526-1530.

Lentjes EG; Griep EN; Boersma JW; Romijn FP; de Kloet ER. (1997). Glucocorticoid receptors, fibromyalgia and low back pain. *Psychoneuroendocrinology* 22(8):603-614.

Maes M; Lin A; Bonaccorso S; van Hunsel F; Van Gastel A; Delmeire L; Biondi M; Bosmans E; Kenis G; Scharpe S. (1998). Increased 24-hour urinary cortisol excretion in patients with post-traumatic stress disorder and patients with major depression, but not in patients with fibromyalgia. *Acta Psychiatrica Scandinavica* 98(4):328-335.

Millea PJ; Holloway RL. (2000). Treating fibromyalgia. *American Family Physician* 62(7):1575-1582, 1587.

Morand EF; Cooley H; Leech M; Littlejohn GO. (1996). Advances in the understanding of neuroendocrine function in rheumatic disease. *Australian and New Zealand Journal of Medicine* 26(4):543-551.

Neeck G. (2000). Neuroendocrine and hormonal perturbations and relations to the serotonergic system in fibromyalgia patients. *Scandinavian Journal of Rheumatology* (Suppl. 113):8-12.

Neeck G; Riedel W. (1999). Hormonal pertubations in fibromyalgia syndrome. *Annals of the New York Academy of Sciences* 876:325-338; discussion 339.

Netter P; Hennig J. (1998). The fibromyalgia syndrome as a manifestation of neuroticism? *Zeitschrift Rheumatologie* 57 (Suppl. 2):105-108.

Ostensen M; Rugelsjoen A; Wigers SH. (1997). The effect of reproductive events and alterations of sex hormone levels on the symptoms of fibromyalgia. *Scandinavian Journal of Rheumatology* 26(5):355-360.

Oye I; Morland LM; Gustafsson H. (1996). [Fibromyalgia and central sensitization] Fibromyalgi og sentral sensitivisering. *Lakartidningen* 93(21):2040.

Pillemer SR; Bradley LA; Crofford LJ; Moldofsky H; Chrousos GP. (1997). The neuroscience and endocrinology of fibromyalgia. *Arthritis and Rheumatism* 40(11):1928-1939.

Raphael KG; Marbach JJ. (2000). Comorbid fibromyalgia accounts for reduced fecundity in women with myofascial face pain. *Clinical Journal of Pain* 16(1): 29-36.

Riedel W; Layka H; Neeck G. (1998). Secretory pattern of GH, TSH, thyroid hormones, ACTH, cortisol, FSH, and LH in patients with fibromyalgia syndrome following systemic injection of the relevant hypothalamic-releasing hormones. *Zeitschrift Rheumatologie* 57 (Suppl. 2):81-87.

Russell IJ. (1998). Neurochemical pathogenesis of fibromyalgia. *Zeitschrift Rheumatologie* 57 (Suppl. 2):63-66.

Samborski W; Stratz T; Schochat T; Mennet P; Muller W. (1996). [Biochemical changes in fibromyalgia] Biochemische veranderungen bei der fibromyalgie. *Zeitschrift Rheumatologie* 55(3):168-173.

Scott LV; Dinan TG. (1999). The neuroendocrinology of chronic fatigue syndrome: Focus on the hypothalamic-pituitary-adrenal axis. *Functional Neurology* 14(1):3-11.

Stanton T. (1999). Coping with stress on the job. *Nursing in New Zealand* 4(11): 17-18.

Torpy DJ; Chrousos GP. (1996). The three-way interactions between the hypothalamic-pituitary-adrenal and gonadal axes and the immune system. *Baillieres Clinical Rheumatology* 10(2):181-198.

Torpy DJ; Papanicolaou DA; Lotsikas AJ; Wilder RL; Chrousos GP; Pillemer SR. (2000). Responses of the sympathetic nervous system and the hypothalamic-pituitary-adrenal axis to interleukin-6: A pilot study in fibromyalgia. *Arthritis and Rheumatism* 43(4):872-880.

Winfield JB. (1999). Pain in fibromyalgia. *Rheumatic Diseases Clinics of North America* 25(1):55-79.

*Neurogenic Inflammation*

Enestrom S; Bengtsson A; Frodin T. (1997). Dermal IgG deposits and increase of mast cells in patients with fibromyalgia—relevant findings or epiphenomena? *Scandinavian Journal of Rheumatology* 26(4):308-313.

*Neuroimaging*

Mountz JM; Bradley LA; Modell JG; Alexander RW; Triana-Alexander M; Aaron LA; Stewart KE; Alarcon GS; Mountz JD. (1995). Fibromyalgia in women. Abnormalities of regional cerebral blood flow in the thalamus and the caudate nucleus are associated with low pain threshold levels. *Arthritis and Rheumatism* 38(7):926-938.

San Pedro EC; Mountz JM; Mountz JD; Liu HG; Katholi CR; Deutsch G. (1998). Familial painful restless legs syndrome correlates with pain dependent variation of blood flow to the caudate, thalamus, and anterior cingulate gyrus. *Journal of Rheumatology* 25(11):2270-2275.

Yang J; Kuikka JT; Vanninen E; Kauppinen T; Lansimies E; Patomaki L. (1999). Evaluation of scatter correction using a single isotope for simultaneous emission and transmission data. Phantom and clinical patient studies. *Nuklearmedizin* 38(2):49-55.

## Neuropeptide Y

Anderberg UM; Liu Z; Berglund L; Nyberg F. (1999). Elevated plasma levels of neuropeptide Y in female fibromyalgia patients. *European Journal of Pain* 3(1):19-30.

Crofford LJ; Engleberg NC; Demitrack MA. (1996). Neurohormonal perturbations in fibromyalgia. *Baillieres Clinical Rheumatology* 10(2):365-378.

## Nociceptin

Anderberg UM; Liu Z; Berglund L; Nyberg F. (1998). Plasma levels of nociceptin in female fibromyalgia syndrome patients. *Zeitschrift Rheumatologie* 57 (Suppl. 2):77-80.

## Nonsteroidal Anti-inflammatory Drugs (NSAIDs)

Vachtenheim J. (1995). [Non-steroidal antirheumatic ointments in the treatment of primary periarticular and intramuscular fibrositis] Nesteroidni antirevmatika v mast'ove forme v lecbe prvotni kolemkloubni a nitrosvalove fibrozitidy. *Vnitr Lek* 41(9):609-612.

Wolfe F; Zhao S; Lane N. (2000). Preference for nonsteroidal antiinflammatory drugs over acetaminophen by rheumatic disease patients: A survey of 1,799 patients with osteoarthritis, rheumatoid arthritis, and fibromyalgia. *Arthritis and Rheumatism* 43(2):378-385.

## Nursing

Edmands MS; Hoff LA; Kaylor L; Mower L; Sorrell S. (1999). Bridging gaps between mind, body, and spirit. Healing the whole person. *Journal of Psychosocial Nursing and Mental Health Services* 37(10):35-42.

Ryan S. (1995). Fibromyalgia: What help can nurses give? *Nursing Stand* 9(37): 25-28.

## Omega-3 Fatty Acids

Ozgocmen S; Catal SA; Ardicoglu O; Kamanli A. (2000). Effect of omega-3 fatty acids in the management of fibromyalgia syndrome. *International Journal of Clinical Pharmacology Therapy* 38(7):362-363.

## Opioids

Quang-Cantagrel ND; Wallace MS; Magnuson SK. (2000). Opioid substitution to improve the effectiveness of chronic noncancer pain control: A chart review. *Anesthedia and Analgesia* 90(4):933-937.

Quijada-Carrera J; Valenzuela-Castano A; Povedano-Gomez J; Fernandez-Rodriguez A; Hernanz-Mediano W; Gutierrez-Rubio A; de la Iglesia-Salgado JL; Garcia-Lopez A. (1996). Comparison of tenoxicam and bromazepan in the treatment of fibromyalgia: A randomized, double-blind, placebo-controlled trial. *Pain* 65(2-3):221-225.

## Orofacial Pain

Bailey DR. (1997). Sleep disorders. Overview and relationship to orofacial pain. *Dentistry Clinics of North America* 41(2):189-209.

Heir GM. (1997). Differentiation of orofacial pain related to Lyme disease from other dental and facial pain disorders. *Dentistry Clinics of North America* 41(2):243-258.

## Osteomalacia

Reginato AJ; Falasca GF; Pappu R; McKnight B; Agha A. (1999). Musculoskeletal manifestations of osteomalacia: Report of 26 cases and literature review. *Seminars in Arthritis and Rheumatism* 28(5):287-304.

## Osteoporosis

Dessein PH; Stanwix AE. (2000). Why would fibromyalgia patients have osteoporosis? *Journal of Rheumatology* 27(7):1816-1817.

Swezey RL; Adams J. (1999). Fibromyalgia: A risk factor for osteoporosis. *Journal of Rheumatology* 26(12):2642-2644.

## Pain

Affleck G; Urrows S; Tennen H; Higgins P; Abeles M. (1996). Sequential daily relations of sleep, pain intensity, and attention to pain among women with fibromyalgia. *Pain* 68(2-3):363-368.

Agargun MY; Tekeoglu I; Gunes A; Adak B; Kara H; Ercan M. (1999). Sleep quality and pain threshold in patients with fibromyalgia. *Comprehensive Psychiatry* 40(3):226-228.

Alvarez-Lario B; Alonso Valdivielso JL; Alegre Lopez J. (1999). [Pathophysiology of pain in fibromyalgia syndrome: On the threshold of its understanding] Fisiopatologia del dolor en el sindrome de fibromialgia: En el umbral de su comprension. *Medicina Clinica* (Barc) 112(16):621-630.

Arner S; Gustafsson L; Hansson P; Kinnman E; Sollevi A; Sorensen J. (1998). [Pharmacological pain analysis as diagnostic and therapeutic help] Farmakologisk smartanalys hjalp vid diagnostik och terapival. *Lakartidningen* 95(24): 2824-2828.

Atkins CJ; Zielinski A; Makosinski A. (1995). Palpometry: A novel concept in pain measurement. *Nature Medicine* 1(11):1138-1139.

Bassoe CF. (1997). [Muscle pain or skin pain?] Muskelverk eller hudverk? *Tidsskr Nor Laegeforen* 117(18):2649-2650.

Bendtsen L; Norregaard J; Jensen R; Olesen J. (1997). Evidence of qualitatively altered nociception in patients with fibromyalgia. *Arthritis and Rheumatism* 40(1): 98-102.

Bengtsson A; Henriksson KG. (1996). [Causes of fibromyalgia are both peripheral and central] Fibromyalgins orsaker bade perifera och centrala. *Lakartidningen* 93(3):161-163.

Bennett RM. (1999). Emerging concepts in the neurobiology of chronic pain: Evidence of abnormal sensory processing in fibromyalgia. *Mayo Clinic Proceedings* 74(4):385-398.

Bradley LA; Alarcon GS; Aaron LA; Martin MY; Alberts KR; Sotolongo A. (1997). Abnormal pain perception in patients with fibromyalgia: Comment on the article by Bendtsen et al. *Arthritis and Rheumatism* 40(12):2275-2277.

Drewes AM. (1999). Pain and sleep disturbances with special reference to fibromyalgia and rheumatoid arthritis. *Rheumatology* (Oxford) 38(11):1035-1038.

Ernberg M; Lundeberg T; Kopp S. (2000). Pain and allodynia/hyperalgesia induced by intramuscular injection of serotonin in patients with fibromyalgia and healthy individuals. *Pain* 85(1-2):31-39.

Ferguson RJ; Ahles TA. (1998). Private body consciousness, anxiety and pain symptom reports of chronic pain patients. *Behaviorial Research and Therapy* 36(5):527-535.

Forseth KO; Husby G; Gran JT; Forre O. (1999). Prognostic factors for the development of fibromyalgia in women with self-reported musculoskeletal pain. A prospective study. *Journal of Rheumatology* 26(11):2458-2467.

Friedman MH; Nelson AJ Jr. (1996). Head and neck pain review: Traditional and new perspectives. *Journal of Orthopedics and Sports Physical Therapy* 24(4): 268-278.

Gustafsson M; Gaston-Johansson F. (1996). Pain intensity and health locus of control: A comparison of patients with fibromyalgia syndrome and rheumatoid arthritis. *Patient Education and Counseling* 29(2):179-188.

Henriksson KG; Backman E; Henriksson C; de Laval JH. (1996). Chronic regional muscular pain in women with precise manipulation work. A study of pain characteristics, muscle function, and impact on daily activities. *Scandinavian Journal of Rheumatology* 25(4):213-223.

Houvenagel E. (1999). Mechanisms of pain in fibromyalgia. *Revue de Rhumatism English Edition* 66(2):97-101.

Kosek E; Ekholm J; Hansson P. (1996). Modulation of pressure pain thresholds during and following isometric contraction in patients with fibromyalgia and in healthy controls. *Pain* 64(3):415-423.

Kosek E; Hansson P. (1997). Modulatory influence on somatosensory perception from vibration and heterotopic noxious conditioning stimulation (HNCS) in fibromyalgia patients and healthy subjects. *Pain* 70(1):41-51.

Kramis RC; Roberts WJ; Gillette RG. (1996). Non-nociceptive aspects of persistent musculoskeletal pain. *Journal of Orthopedics and Sports Physical Therapy* 24(4):255-267.

Lautenbacher S; Rollman GB. (1997). Possible deficiencies of pain modulation in fibromyalgia. *Clinical Journal of Pain* 13(3):189-196.

Lidbeck J. (1999). [Centrally disturbed pain modulation explains prolonged pain. New knowledge changes the view on the problematic patient] Centralt stord smartmodulering forklaring till langvarig smarta. Nya kunskaper forandrar synen pa den problematiska smartpatienten. *Lakartidningen* 96(23):2843-2848, 2850-2851.

Lorenz J; Grasedyck K; Bromm B. (1996). Middle and long latency somatosensory evoked potentials after painful laser stimulation in patients with fibromyalgia syndrome. *Electroencephalography and Clinical Neurophysiology* 100(2):165-168.

MacFarlane GJ. (1999). Generalized pain, fibromyalgia and regional pain: An epidemiological view. *Baillieres Best Practice Reseach in Clinical Rheumatology* 13(3):403-414.

MacFarlane GJ; Croft PR; Schollum J; Silman AJ. (1996). Widespread pain: Is an improved classification possible? *Journal of Rheumatology* 23(9):1628-1632.

Morris V; Cruwys S; Kidd B. (1998). Increased capsaicin-induced secondary hyperalgesia as a marker of abnormal sensory activity in patients with fibromyalgia. *Neurosciences Letters* 250(3):205-207.

Mountz JM; Bradley LA; Alarcon GS. (1998). Abnormal functional activity of the central nervous system in fibromyalgia syndrome. *American Journal of Medical Sciences* 315(6):385-396.

Nicassio PM; Schoenfeld-Smith K; Radojevic V; Schuman C. (1995). Pain coping mechanisms in fibromyalgia: Relationship to pain and functional outcomes. *Journal of Rheumatology* 22(8):1552-1558.

Reilly PA. (1999). The differential diagnosis of generalized pain. *Baillieres Best Practice Research in Clinical Rheumatology* 13(3):391-401.

Rubio Montanes ML; Prat Gil N; Adalid Villar C; Pueyo Anton L. (1995). [Prevalence of generalized pain of the locomotor system] Prevalencia del dolor generalizado del aparato locomotor. *Atencion Primaria* 16(6):379-380.

Russell IJ. (1998). Advances in fibromyalgia: Possible role for central neurochemicals. *American Journal of Medical Sciences* 315(6):377-384.

Sartin JS. (2000). Fibromyalgia and pain management. *Mayo Clinic Proceedings* 75(3):316-317.

Schadrack J; Zieglgansberger W. (1998). Pharmacology of pain processing systems. *Zeitschrift Rheumatologie* 57 (Suppl. 2):1-4.

Smythe HA; Gladman A; Mader R; Peloso P; Abu-Shakra M. (1997). Strategies for assessing pain and pain exaggeration: Controlled studies. *Journal of Rheumatology* 24(8):1622-1629.

Sorensen J; Bengtsson A; Ahlner J; Henriksson KG; Ekselius L; Bengtsson M. (1997). Fibromyalgia—are there different mechanisms in the processing of pain? A double blind crossover comparison of analgesic drugs. *Journal of Rheumatology* 24(8):1615-1621.

Sorensen J; Graven-Nielsen T; Henriksson KG; Bengtsson M; Arendt-Nielsen L. (1998). Hyperexcitability in fibromyalgia. *Journal of Rheumatology* 25(1):152-155.

Turk DC; Okifuji A. (1997). Evaluating the role of physical, operant, cognitive, and affective factors in the pain behaviors of chronic pain patients. *Behavior Modification* 21(3):259-280.

Weigent DA; Bradley LA; Blalock JE; Alarcon GS. (1998). Current concepts in the pathophysiology of abnormal pain perception in fibromyalgia. *American Journal of Medical Sciences* 315(6):405-412.

White KP; Harth M. (1999). The occurrence and impact of generalized pain. *Baillieres Best Practice Research in Clinical Rheumatology* 13(3):379-389.

Zetterberg C. (1996). [Unclear pathomechanism behind neck-shoulder pain. Problem with insurance claim] Oklar patomekanism bakom nack—skuldervark. Problem vid forsakringsmedicinsk bedomning. *Lakartidningen* 93(9):793-796.

### Pain Syndromes

Carette S. (1996). Chronic pain syndromes. *Annals of Rheumatic Diseases* 55(8): 497-501.

Gowin KM. (2000). Diffuse pain syndromes in the elderly. *Rheumatic Diseases Clinics of North America* 26(3):673-682.

Hall S. (1999). Common pain scenarios. *Australian Family Physician* 28(1):31-35.

Linaker CH; Walker-Bone K; Palmer K; Cooper C. (1999). Frequency and impact of regional musculoskeletal disorders. *Baillieres Clinical Rheumatology* 13(2): 197-215.

MacFarlane GJ; Thomas E; Papageorgiou AC; Schollum J; Croft PR; Silman AJ. (1996). The natural history of chronic pain in the community: A better prognosis than in the clinic? *Journal of Rheumatology* 23(9):1617-1620.

Menninger H. (1998). Other pain syndromes to be differentiated from fibromyalgia. *Zeitschrift Rheumatologie* 57 (Suppl. 2):56-60.

### Pentazocine-Induced Fibrous Myopathy

Sinsawaiwong S; Phanthumchinda K. (1998). Pentazocine-induced fibrous myopathy and localized neuropathy. *Journal of the Medical Association of Thailand* 81(9):717-721.

## Persian Gulf War Syndrome

Alloway JA; Older SA; Battafarano DF; Carpenter MT. (1998). Persian Gulf War myalgia syndrome. *Journal of Rheumatology* 25(2):388-389.

Escalante A; Fischbach M. (1998). Musculoskeletal manifestations, pain, and quality of life in Persian Gulf War veterans referred for rheumatologic evaluation. *Journal of Rheumatology* 25(11):2228-2235.

Grady EP; Carpenter MT; Koenig CD; Older SA; Battafarano DF. (1998). Rheumatic findings in Gulf War veterans. *Archives of Internal Medicine* 158(4):367-371.

Hodgson MJ; Kipen HM. (1999). Gulf War illnesses: Causation and treatment. *Journal of Occupational and Environmental Medicine* 41(6):443-452.

Nicolson GL; Nicolson NL. (1998). Gulf War illnesses: Complex medical, scientific and political paradox. *Medicine of Conflict Survivors* 14(2):156-165.

Self-reported illness and health status among Gulf War veterans: A population-based study. The Iowa Persian Gulf Study Group. (1997). *Journal of the American Medical Association* 277(3):238-245.

Smith TC; Gray GC; Knoke JD. (2000). Is systemic lupus erythematosus, amyotrophic lateral sclerosis, or fibromyalgia associated with Persian Gulf War service? An examination of Department of Defense hospitalization data. *American Journal of Epidemiology* 151(11):1053-1059.

## Phenobarbital

Goldman SI; Krings MS. (1995). Phenobarbital-induced fibromyalgia as the cause of bilateral shoulder pain. *Journal of the American Osteopathic Association* 95(8):487-490.

## Phosphate Diabetes

De Lorenzo F; Hargreaves J; Kakkar VV. (1998). Phosphate diabetes in patients with chronic fatigue syndrome. *Postgraduate Medical Journal* 74(870):229-232.

Laroche M; Tack Y. (1999). Hypophosphoremia secondary to idiopathic moderate phosphate diabetes: A differential diagnosis with primary fibromyalgia. *Clinical and Experimental Rheumatology* 17(5):628.

## Physical Therapy

Mengshoel AM. (1997). [Physical therapy and fibromyalgia] Fysioterapi og fibromyalgi. *Tidsskr Nor Laegeforen* 117(30):4484-4485.

Offenbacher M; Stucki G. (2000). Physical therapy in the treatment of fibromyalgia. *Scandinavian Journal of Rheumatology* (Suppl. 113):78-85.

### Platelet Alpha-2-Adrenoreceptors

Maes M; Libbrecht I; Delmeire L; Lin A; De Clerck L; Scharpe S; Janca A. (1999). Changes in platelet alpha-2-adrenoceptors in fibromyalgia: Effects of treatment with antidepressants. *Neuropsychobiology* 40(3):129-133.

### Polymyalgia Rheumatica

Nishikai M. (1999). [Polymyalgia rheumatica]. *Nippon Rinsho* 57(2):370-373.

### Postcardiac Injury Rheumatism

Mukhopadhyay P; Chakraborty S; Mukherjee S. (1995). Postcardiac injury rheumatism. *Journal of the Association of Physicians of India* 43(6):388-90.

### Post-Lyme Disease Syndrome

Berman DS; Wenglin BD. (1995). Complaints attributed to chronic Lyme disease: Depression or fibromyalgia? *American Journal of Medicine* 99(4):440.

Bujak DI; Weinstein A; Dornbush RL. (1996). Clinical and neurocognitive features of the post Lyme syndrome. *Journal of Rheumatology* 23(8):1392-1397.

Ellenbogen C. (1997). Lyme disease. Shift the paradigm! *Archives of Family Medicine* 6(2):191-195.

Fallon J; Bujak DI; Guardino S; Weinstein A. (1999). The Fibromyalgia Impact Questionnaire: A useful tool in evaluating patients with post-Lyme disease syndrome. *Arthritis Care Research* 12(1):42-47.

Frey M; Jaulhac B; Piemont Y; Marcellin L; Boohs PM; Vautravers P; Jesel M; Kuntz JL; Monteil H; Sibilia J. (1998). Detection of *Borrelia burgdorferi* DNA in muscle of patients with chronic myalgia related to Lyme disease. *American Journal of Medicine* 104(6):591-594.

Frey M; Jaulhac B; Sibilia J; Monteil H; Kuntz JL; Vautravers P. (1995). [Detection of *Borrelia burgdorferi* DNA by gene amplification in the muscle of a patient with fibromyalgia] Detection d'ADN de *Borrelia burgdorferi* par amplification genique dans le muscle d'un patient atteint de fibromyalgie. *Presse Medicale* 24(34):1623.

Graninger W. (1996). A "minority" opinion about the diagnosis and treatment of Lyme arthritis. *Infection* 24(1):95-97.

Nadelman RB; Nowakowski J; Wormser GP; Schwartz I. (1999). How should viability of *Borrelia burgdorferi* be demonstrated? *American Journal of Medicine* 106(4):491-492.

Rahn DW; Felz MW. (1998). Lyme disease update. Current approach to early, disseminated, and late disease. *Postgraduate Medicine* 103(5):51-54, 57-59, 63-64 passim.

Sigal LH. (1995). Diagnosis of Lyme disease. *Journal of the American Medical Association* 274(18):1427-1428.

## Postpolio Syndrome

Trojan DA; Cashman NR. (1995). Fibromyalgia is common in a postpoliomyelitis clinic. *Archives of Neurology* 52(6):620-624.

## Post-Traumatic Stress Disorder

Amir M; Kaplan Z; Neumann L; Sharabani R; Shani N; Buskila D. (1997). Posttraumatic stress disorder, tenderness and fibromyalgia. *Journal of Psychosomatic Research* 42(6):607-613.

Sherman JJ; Turk DC; Okifuji A. (2000). Prevalence and impact of posttraumatic stress disorder-like symptoms on patients with fibromyalgia syndrome. *Clinical Journal of Pain* 16(2):127-134.

## Propyl Endopeptidase

Maes M; Libbrecht I; Van Hunsel F; Lin AH; Bonaccorso S; Goossens F; De Meester I; De Clerck L; Biondi M; Scharpe S; Janca A. (1998). Lower serum activity of prolyl endopeptidase in fibromyalgia is related to severity of depressive symptoms and pressure hyperalgesia. *Psychological Medicine* 28(4):957-965.

## Prostaglandin D Synthase

Melegos DN; Freedman MS; Diamandis EP. (1997). Prostaglandin D synthase concentration in cerebrospinal fluid and serum of patients with neurological disorders. *Prostaglandins* 54(1):463-474.

## Protein Peroxidation

Eisinger J; Zakarian H; Pouly E; Plantamura A; Ayavou T. (1996). Protein peroxidation, magnesium deficiency and fibromyalgia. *Magnesium Research* 9(4):313-316.

## Psychiatry

Aaron LA; Bradley LA; Alarcon GS; Alexander RW; Triana-Alexander M; Martin MY; Alberts KR. (1996). Psychiatric diagnoses in patients with fibromyalgia are related to health care-seeking behavior rather than to illness. *Arthritis and Rheumatism* 39(3):436-445.

Avina-Zubieta JA; Paez F; Galindo-Rodriguez G. (1997). Rheumatic manifestations of neurologic and psychiatric diseases. *Current Opinions in Rheumatology* 9(1):51-55.

Benjamin S; Morris S; McBeth J; Macfarlane GJ; Silman AJ. (2000). The association between chronic widespread pain and mental disorder: A population-based study. *Arthritis and Rheumatism* 43(3):561-567.

Ben-Zion I; Shieber A; Buskila D. (1996). [Psychiatric aspects of fibromyalgia syndrome]. *Harefuah* 131(3-4):127-129.

Dunne FJ; Dunne CA. (1995). Fibromyalgia syndrome and psychiatric disorder. *British Journal of Hospital Medicine* 54(5):194-197.

Epstein SA; Kay G; Clauw D; Heaton R; Klein D; Krupp L; Kuck J; Leslie V; Masur D; Wagner M; Waid R; Zisook S. (1999). Psychiatric disorders in patients with fibromyalgia. A multicenter investigation. *Psychosomatics* 40(1):57-63.

Gruber AJ; Hudson JI; Pope HG Jr. (1996). The management of treatment-resistant depression in disorders on the interface of psychiatry and medicine. Fibromyalgia, chronic fatigue syndrome, migraine, irritable bowel syndrome, atypical facial pain, and premenstrual dysphoric disorder. *Psychiatry Clinics of North America* 19(2):351-369.

Hudson JI; Pope HG Jr. (1996). The relationship between fibromyalgia and major depressive disorder. *Rheumatic Diseases Clinics of North America* 22(2):285-303.

Katz RS; Kravitz HM. (1996). Fibromyalgia, depression, and alcoholism: A family history study. *Journal of Rheumatology* 23(1):149-154.

Keel P. (1998). Psychological and psychiatric aspects of fibromyalgia syndrome (FMS). *Zeitschrift Rheumatologie* 57 (Suppl. 2):97-100.

Meyer-Lindenberg A; Gallhofer B. (1998). Somatized depression as a subgroup of fibromyalgia syndrome. *Zeitschrift Rheumatologie* 57 (Suppl. 2):92-93.

Offenbaecher M; Glatzeder K; Ackenheil M. (1998). Self-reported depression, familial history of depression and fibromyalgia (FM), and psychological distress in patients with FM. *Zeitschrift Rheumatologie* 57 (Suppl. 2):94-96.

Ruderman EM; Golden HE. (1996). Psychiatric diagnoses in patients with fibromyalgia: Comment on the article by Aaron et al. *Arthritis and Rheumatism* 39(12):2086-2087.

*Psychosocial Factors*

Affleck G; Tennen H; Urrows S; Higgins P; Abeles M; Hall C; Karoly P; Newton C. (1998). Fibromyalgia and women's pursuit of personal goals: A daily process analysis. *Health Psychology* 17(1):40-47.

Anderberg UM. (1999). [Stress can induce neuroendocrine disorders and pain] Stress kan ge neuroendokrina storningar och smarttillstand. *Lakartidningen* 96(49):5497-5499.

Eich W; Hartmann M; Muller A; Fischer H. (2000). The role of psychosocial factors in fibromyalgia syndrome. *Scandinavian Journal of Rheumatology* (Suppl. 113): 30-31.

Hallberg LR; Carlsson SG. (1998). Psychosocial vulnerability and maintaining forces related to fibromyalgia. In-depth interviews with twenty-two female patients. *Scandinavian Journal of Caring Sciences* 12(2):95-103.

Jamison JR. (1999a). A psychological profile of fibromyalgia patients: A chiropractic case study. *Journal of Manipulative Physiology Therapy* 22(7):454-457.

Jamison JR. (1999b). Stress: The chiropractic patients' self-perceptions. *Journal of Manipulative Physiology Therapy* 22(6):395-398.

Neumann L; Buskila D. (1998). Ethnocultural and educational differences in Israeli women correlate with pain perception in fibromyalgia. *Journal of Rheumatology* 25(7):1369-1373.

Rosenfeld WD; Walco GA. (1997). One test too many: Toward an integrated approach to psychosomatic disorders. *Adolescent Medicine* 8(3):483-487.

Turk DC; Okifuji A; Sinclair JD; Starz TW. (1998). Differential responses by psychosocial subgroups of fibromyalgia syndrome patients to an interdisciplinary treatment. *Arthritis Care Research* 11(5):397-404.

Walker EA; Keegan D; Gardner G; Sullivan M; Katon WJ; Bernstein D. (1997). Psychosocial factors in fibromyalgia compared with rheumatoid arthritis: I. Psychiatric diagnoses and functional disability. *Psychosomatic Medicine* 59(6):565-571.

Wolfe F; Hawley DJ. (1998). Psychosocial factors and the fibromyalgia syndrome. *Zeitschrift Rheumatologie* 57 (Suppl. 2):88-91.

*Quality of Life*

Buskila D; Zaks N; Neumann L; Livneh A; Greenberg S; Pras M; Langevitz P. (1997). Quality of life of patients with familial Mediterranean fever. *Clinical and Experimental Rheumatology* 15(4):355-360.

Kurtze N; Gundersen KT; Svebak S. (1999). Quality of life, functional disability and lifestyle among subgroups of fibromyalgia patients: The significance of anxiety and depression. *British Journal of Medical Psychology* 72(Pt. 4):471-484.

Neumann L; Buskila D. (1997). Quality of life and physical functioning of relatives of fibromyalgia patients. *Seminars in Arthritis and Rheumatism* 26(6):834-839.

Ruiz Moral R; Munoz Alamo M; Perula de Torres L; Aguayo Galeote M. (1997). Biopsychosocial features of patients with widespread chronic musculoskeletal pain in family medicine clinics. *Family Practice* 14(3):242-248.

Schlenk EA; Erlen JA; Dunbar-Jacob J; McDowell J; Engberg S; Sereika SM; Rohay JM; Bernier MJ. (1998). Health-related quality of life in chronic disorders: a comparison across studies using the MOS SF-36. *Quality of Life Research* 7(1):57-65.

Soderberg S; Lundman B; Norberg A. (1997). Living with fibromyalgia: Sense of coherence, perception of well-being, and stress in daily life. *Research on Nursing and Health* 20(6):495-503.

Strombeck B; Ekdahl C; Manthorpe R; Wikstrom I; Jacobsson L. (2000). Health-related quality of life in primary Sjogren's syndrome, rheumatoid arthritis and fibromyalgia compared to normal population data using SF-36. *Scandinavian Journal of Rheumatology* 29(1):20-28.

Wolfe F; Hawley DJ. (1997). Measurement of the quality of life in rheumatic disorders using the EuroQol. *British Journal of Rheumatology* 36(7):786-793.

### Raynaud's Phenomenon

Grassi W; De Angelis R; Lapadula G; Leardini G; Scarpa R. (1998). Clinical diagnosis found in patients with Raynaud's phenomenon: A multicentre study. *Rheumatology International* 18(1):17-20.

### Rehabilitation

Berg JE; Berg O; Reiten T; Kostveit S. (1998). Functional diagnosis as a tool in rehabilitation: A comparison of teachers and other employees. *International Journal of Rehabilitation Research* 21(3):273-284.

Buckelew SP; Huyser B; Hewett JE; Parker JC; Johnson JC; Conway R; Kay DR. (1996). Self-efficacy predicting outcome among fibromyalgia subjects. *Arthritis Care Research* 9(2):97-104.

Epifanov VA; Epifanov AV. (2000). [Methods of physical rehabilitation in fibromyalgia] Metody fizicheskoi reabilitatsii pri fibromialgii. *Vopr Kurortol Fizioter Lech Fiz Kult* (3):42-45.

Karjalainen K; Malmivaara A; van Tulder M; Roine R; Jauhiainen M; Hurri H; Koes B. (2000). Multidisciplinary rehabilitation for fibromyalgia and musculoskeletal pain in working age adults. *Cochrane Database Systematic Review* (2):CD001984.

### Rhinitis

Baraniuk JN; Clauw D; Yuta A; Ali M; Gaumond E; Upadhyayula N; Fujita K; Shimizu T. (1998). Nasal secretion analysis in allergic rhinitis, cystic fibrosis, and nonallergic fibromyalgia/chronic fatigue syndrome subjects. *American Journal of Rhinology* 12(6):435-440.

Baraniuk JN; Naranch K; Maibach H; Clauw D. (2000). Irritant rhinitis in allergic, nonallergic, control and chronic fatigue syndrome populations. *Journal of Chronic Fatigue Syndrome* 7(2):3-32.

### Ritanserin

Olin R; Klein R; Berg PA. (1998). A randomised double-blind 16-week study of ritanserin in fibromyalgia syndrome: Clinical outcome and analysis of autoantibodies to serotonin, gangliosides and phospholipids. *Clinical Rheumatology* 17(2):89-94.

### Rubella Vaccines

Weibel RE; Benor DE. (1996). Chronic arthropathy and musculoskeletal symptoms associated with rubella vaccines. A review of 124 claims submitted to the National Vaccine Injury Compensation Program. *Arthritis and Rheumatism* 39(9):1529-1534.

## S-adenosyl-L-methionine

Tavoni A; Jeracitano G; Cirigliano G. (1998). Evaluation of S-adenosylmethionine in secondary fibromyalgia: a double-blind study. *Clinical and Experimental Rheumatology* 16(1):106-107.

Volkmann H; Norregaard J; Jacobsen S; Danneskiold-Samsoe B; Knoke G; Nehrdich D. (1997). Double-blind, placebo-controlled cross-over study of intravenous S-adenosyl-L-methionine in patients with fibromyalgia. *Scandinavian Journal of Rheumatology* 26(3):206-211.

## Saliva

Fischer HP; Eich W; Russell IJ. (1998). A possible role for saliva as a diagnostic fluid in patients with chronic pain. *Seminars in Arthritis and Rheumatism* 27(6):348-359.

## Sarcoid Arthritis

Gran JT; Bohmer E. (1996). Acute sarcoid arthritis: a favourable outcome? A retrospective survey of 49 patients with review of the literature. *Scandinavian Journal of Rheumatology* 25(2):70-73.

## Scleritis

Fan NI; Florakis GJ. (1996). Scleritis associated with the fibromyalgia syndrome. *Cornea* 15(6):637-638.

## Selective Serotonin Reuptake Inhibitors (Fluoxetine, Citalopram)

Anderberg UM; Marteinsdottir I; von Knorring L. (2000). Citalopram in patients with fibromyalgia—a randomized, double-blind, placebo-controlled study. *European Journal of Pain* 4(1):27-35.

Chambliss ML. (1998). Are serotonin uptake inhibitors useful in chronic pain syndromes such as fibromyalgia or diabetic neuropathy? *Archives of Family Medicine* 7(5):470-471.

Goldenberg D; Mayskiy M; Mossey C; Ruthazer R; Schmid C. (1996). A randomized, double-blind crossover trial of fluoxetine and amitriptyline in the treatment of fibromyalgia. *Arthritis and Rheumatism* 39(11):1852-1859.

Jung AC; Staiger T; Sullivan M. (1997). The efficacy of selective serotonin reuptake inhibitors for the management of chronic pain. *Journal of General Internal Medicine* 12(6):384-389.

Nerhood RC. (1998). Fluoxetine and pregnancy a safe mix? *Postgraduate Medicine* 104(5):37-38.

Norregaard J; Volkmann H; Danneskiold-Samsoe B. (1995). A randomized controlled trial of citalopram in the treatment of fibromyalgia. *Pain* 61(3):445-449.

Smith AJ. (1998). The analgesic effects of selective serotonin reuptake inhibitors. *Journal of Psychopharmacology* 12(4):407-413.

## Selenium

Reinhard P; Schweinsberg F; Wernet D; Kotter I. (1998). Selenium status in fibromyalgia. *Toxicology Letters* 96-97:177-180.

## Self-Esteem

Johnson M; Paananen ML; Rahinantti P; Hannonen P. (1997). Depressed fibromyalgia patients are equipped with an emphatic competence dependent self-esteem. *Clinical Rheumatology* 16(6):578-584.

## Serotonin

Ernberg M; Hedenberg-Magnusson B; Alstergren P; Kopp S. (1998). Effect of local glucocorticoid injection on masseter muscle level of serotonin in patients with chronic myalgia. *Acta Odontologica Scandinavica* 56(3):129-134.

Ernberg M; Hedenberg-Magnusson B; Alstergren P; Kopp S. (1999). The level of serotonin in the superficial masseter muscle in relation to local pain and allodynia. *Life Sciences* 65(3):313-325.

Ernberg M; Hedenberg-Magnusson B; Alstergren P; Lundeberg T; Kopp S. (1999). Pain, allodynia, and serum serotonin level in orofacial pain of muscular origin. *Journal of Orofacial Pain* 13(1):56-62.

Juhl JH. (1998). Fibromyalgia and the serotonin pathway. *Alternative Medicine Reviews* 3(5):367-375.

Nicolodi M; Volpe AR; Sicuteri F. (1998). Fibromyalgia and headache. Failure of serotonergic analgesia and N-methyl-D-aspartate-mediated neuronal plasticity: their common clues. *Cephalalgia* 18 (Suppl. 21):41-44.

Sprott H; Bradley LA; Oh SJ; Wintersberger W; Alarcon GS; Mussell HG; Tseng A; Gay RE; Gay S. (1998). Immunohistochemical and molecular studies of serotonin, substance P, galanin, pituitary adenylyl cyclase-activating polypeptide, and secretoneurin in fibromyalgic muscle tissue. *Arthritis and Rheumatism* 41(9):1689-1694.

Wolfe F; Russell IJ; Vipraio G; Ross K; Anderson J. (1997). Serotonin levels, pain threshold, and fibromyalgia symptoms in the general population. *Journal of Rheumatology* 24(3):555-559.

## Serotonin 3-Receptor Antagonists (Tropisetron, Ondansetron)

Farber L; Stratz T; Bruckle W; Spath M; Pongratz D; Lautenschlager J; Kotter I; Zoller B; Peter HH; Neeck G; Alten R; Muller W. (2000). Efficacy and tolerability of tropisetron in primary fibromyalgia—a highly selective and competitive 5-HT3 receptor antagonist. German Fibromyalgia Study Group. *Scandinavian Journal of Rheumatology* (Suppl. 113):49-54.

Haus U; Varga B; Stratz T; Spath M; Muller W. (2000). Oral treatment of fibromyalgia with tropisetron given over 28 days: Influence on functional and vegetative symptoms, psychometric parameters and pain. *Scandinavian Journal of Rheumatology* (Suppl. 113):55-58.

Hocherl K; Farber L; Ladenburger S; Vosshage D; Stratz T; Muller W; Grobecker H. (2000). Effect of tropisetron on circulating catecholamines and other putative biochemical markers in serum of patients with fibromyalgia. *Scandinavian Journal of Rheumatology* (Suppl. 113):46-48.

Hrycaj P; Stratz T; Mennet P; Muller W. (1996). Pathogenetic aspects of responsiveness to ondansetron (5-hydroxytryptamine type 3 receptor antagonist) in patients with primary fibromyalgia syndrome—a preliminary study. *Journal of Rheumatology* 23(8):1418-1423.

Muller W; Stratz T. (2000). Results of the intravenous administration of tropisetron in fibromyalgia patients. *Scandinavian Journal of Rheumatology* (Suppl. 113):59-62.

Papadopoulos IA; Georgiou PE; Katsimbri PP; Drosos AA. (2000). Treatment of fibromyalgia with tropisetron, a 5HT3 serotonin antagonist: A pilot study. *Clinical Rheumatology* 19(1):6-8.

Samborski W; Stratz T; Lacki JK; Klama K; Mennet P; Muller W. (1996). The 5-HT3 blockers in the treatment of the primary fibromyalgia syndrome: A 10-day open study with Tropisetron at a low dose. *Mater Medica Polaca* 28(1):17-19.

Stratz T; Muller W. (2000a). Do predictors exist for the therapeutic effect of 5-HT3 receptor antagonists in fibromyalgia? *Scandinavian Journal of Rheumatology* (Suppl. 113):63-65.

Stratz T; Muller W. (2000b). The use of 5-HT3 receptor antagonists in various rheumatic diseases—a clue to the mechanism of action of these agents in fibromyalgia? *Scandinavian Journal of Rheumatology* (Suppl. 113):66-71.

Wolf H. (2000). Preclinical and clinical pharmacology of the 5-HT3 receptor antagonists. *Scandinavian Journal of Rheumatology* (Suppl. 113):37-45.

*Serotonin Receptor Gene*

Bondy B; Spaeth M; Offenbaecher M; Glatzeder K; Stratz T; Schwarz M; de Jonge S; Kruger M; Engel RR; Farber L; Pongratz DE; Ackenheil M. (1999). The T102C polymorphism of the 5-HT2A-receptor gene in fibromyalgia. *Neurobiological Diseases* 6(5):433-439.

*Serotonin Transporter Gene*

Offenbaecher M; Bondy B; de Jonge S; Glatzeder K; Kruger M; Schoeps P; Ackenheil M. (1999). Possible association of fibromyalgia with a polymorphism in the serotonin transporter gene regulatory region. *Arthritis and Rheumatism* 42(11):2482-2488.

## Serum Nucleotide Pyrophosphohydrolase

Cardenal A; Masuda I; Ono W; Haas AL; Ryan LM; Trotter D; McCarty DJ. (1998). Serum nucleotide pyrophosphohydrolase activity; elevated levels in osteoarthritis, calcium pyrophosphate crystal deposition disease, scleroderma, and fibromyalgia. *Journal of Rheumatology* 25(11):2175-2180.

## Sjogren's Syndrome

Dohrenbusch R; Gruterich M; Genth E. (1996). [Fibromyalgia and Sjogren syndrome—clinical and methodological aspects] Fibromyalgie und Sjogren-syndrom—klinische und methodische aspekte. *Zeitschrift Rheumatologie* 55(1):19-27.

Fox RI. (1997). Sjogren's syndrome. Controversies and progress. *Clinical Laboratory Medicine* 17(3):431-444.

Fox RI; Stern M; Michelson P. (2000). Update in Sjogren syndrome. *Current Opinions in Rheumatology* 12(5):391-398.

Fox RI; Tornwall J; Maruyama T; Stern M. (1998). Evolving concepts of diagnosis, pathogenesis, and therapy of Sjogren's syndrome. *Current Opinions in Rheumatology* 10(5):446-456.

Giles I; Isenberg D. (2000). Fatigue in primary Sjogren's syndrome: Is there a link with the fibromyalgia syndrome? *Annals of Rheumatic Diseases* 59(11):875-878.

## Skinache Syndrome

Bassoe CF. (1995). The skinache syndrome. *Journal of the Royal Society of Medicine* 88(10):565-569.

## Sleep

Affleck G; Urrows S; Tennen H; Higgins O; Abeles M. (1996). Sequential daily relations of sleep, pain intensity, and attention to pain among women with fibromyalgia. *Pain* 68:363-368.

Agargun MY; Tekeoglu I; Gunes A; Adak B; Kara H; Ercan M. (1999). Sleep quality and pain threshold in patients with fibromyalgia. *Comprehensive Psychiatry* 40(3):226-228.

Alvarez-Lario B; Alonso Valdivielso JL; Alegre Lopez J; Martel Soteres C; Viejo Banuelos JL; Maranon Cabello A. (1996). Fibromyalgia syndrome: Overnight falls in arterial oxygen saturation. *American Journal of Medicine* 101(1):54-60.

Anch AM; Lue FA; MacLean AW; Moldofsky H. (1991). Sleep physiology and psychological aspects of fibrositis (fibromyalgia) syndrome. *Canadian Journal of Experimental Psychology* 45:179-184.

Atkinson JH; Ancoli-Israel S; Slater MA; Garfin SR; Gillin JC. (1988). Subjective sleep disturbances in chronic back pain. *Clinical Journal of Pain* 4:225-232.

Branco J, Atalaia A; Paiva T. (1994). Sleep cycles and alpha-delta sleep in fibromyalgia syndrome. *Journal of Rheumatology* 21:1113-1117.

Campbell SM; Clark S; Tindall EA; Forehand ME; Bennett RM. (1983). Clinical characteristics of fibrositis. I. A "blinded," controlled study of symptoms and tender points. *Arthritis and Rheumatism* 26:817-824.

Clauw D; Blank C; Hiltz R; Katz P; Potolicchio S. (1994). Polysomnography in fibromyalgia patients. *Arthritis and Rheumatism* 37 (Suppl. 9):S348.

Côte KA; Moldofsky H. (1997). Sleep, daytime symptoms, and cognitive performance in patients with fibromyalgia. *Journal of Rheumatology* 24(10):2014-2023.

Croft P; Schollum J; Silman A. (1994). Population study of tender point counts and pain as evidence of fibromyalgia. *British Medical Journal* 309:696-699.

Donald F; Esdaile JM; Kimoff JR; Fitzcharles MA. (1996). Musculoskeletal complaints and fibromyalgia in patients attending a respiratory sleep disorders clinic. *Journal of Rheumatology* 23(9):1612-1616.

Drewes AM; Gade K; Nielsen KD; Bjerregard K; Taagholt SJ; Svendsen L. (1995). Clustering of sleep electroencephalographic patterns in patients with the fibromyalgia syndrome. *British Journal of Rheumatology* 34(12):1151-1156.

Drewes AM; Nielsen KD; Taagholt SJ; Bjerregard K; Svendsen L; Gade J. (1995). Sleep intensity in fibromyalgia: Focus on the microstructure of the sleep process. *British Journal of Rheumatology* 34(7):629-635.

Drewes AM; Nielsen KD; Taagholt SJ; Svendsen L; Bjerregard K; Nielsson L; Kristensen L. (1996). Ambulatory polysomnography using a new programmable amplifier system with on-line digitization of data: Technical and clinical findings. *Sleep* 19(4):347-54.

Fischler B; Le Bon O; Hoffmann G; Cluydts R; Kaufman L; De Meirleir K. (1997). Sleep anomalies in the chronic fatigue syndrome. A comorbidity study. *Neuropsychobiology* 35(3):115-122.

Flanigan MJ; Morehouse RL; Shapiro CM. (1995). Determination of observer-rated alpha activity during sleep. *Sleep* 18(8):702-706.

Green S. (1999). Sleep cycles, TMD, fibromyalgia, and their relationship to orofacial myofunctional disorders. *International Journal of Orofacial Myology* 25:4-14.

Greenberg HE; Ney G; Ravdin L; Scharf SM; Hilton E. (1995). Sleep quality in Lyme disease. *Sleep* 18:912-916.

Hansotia P. (1996). Emotional distress, physical symptoms and sleep disorders. *Wisconsin Medical Journal* 95(12):836-837.

Harding SM. (1998). Sleep in fibromyalgia patients: Subjective and objective findings. *American Journal of Medical Sciences* 315(6):367-376.

Hemmeter U; Kocher R; Ladewig D; Hatzinger M; Seifritz E; Lauer CJ; Holsboer-Trachsler E. (1995). [Sleep disorders in chronic pain and generalized tendomyopathy] Schlafstorungen bei chronischen schmerzen und generalisierter tendomyopathie. *Schweize Medizin Wochenschrift* 125(49):2391-2397.

Hench PK. (1996). Sleep and rheumatic diseases. *Bulletin of Rheumatic Diseases* 45:1-6.

Hirsch M; Carlander B; Verge M; Tafti M; Anaya J-M; Billiard M; Sany J. (1994). Objective and subjective sleep disturbances in patients with rheumatoid arthritis: A reappraisal. *Arthritis and Rheumatism* 37:41-49.

Horne JA; Shackeel BS. (1991). Alpha-like EEG activity in non-REM sleep and the fibromyalgia (fibrositis) syndrome. *Electroencephalographic and Clinical Neurophysiology* 79:271-276.

Hyyppa MT; Kronholm E. (1995). Nocturnal motor activity in fibromyalgia patients with poor sleep quality. *Journal of Psychosomatic Research* 39:85-91.

Kempenaers C; Simenon G; Elst MV; Fransolet L; Mingard P; de Maertelaer V; Appelboom T; Mendlewicz J. (1994). Effect of antidiencephalon immune serum on pain and sleep in primary fibromyalgia. *Neuropsychobiology* 30:66-72.

Kryeger JM. (1995). Cytokines and sleep. *International Archives of Allergy and Immunology* 106:97-100.

Kryger M; Shapiro CM. (1992). Pain and distress at night. *Sleep Solutions* 5:1-20.

Leigh TJ; Hindmarch I; Bird HA; Wright V. (1998). Comparison of sleep in osteoarthritis patients and age-sex matched healthy controls. *Annals of Rheumatic Diseases* 47:40-42.

Lentz MJ; Landis CA; Rothermel J; Shaver JL. (1999). Effects of selective slow wave sleep disruption on musculoskeletal pain and fatigue in middle aged women. *Journal of Rheumatology* 26(7):1586-1592.

Lugaresi E; Cirignotta F; Zucconi M; Mondini S; Lenzi PL; Coccagna G. (1981). Good and poor sleepers: An epidemiological survey of the San Marino population. In Guilleminault C; Lugareso E, editors. *Sleep/wake disorders: Natural history.* New York: Raven Press; pp.1-12.

MacFarlane JG; Shahal B; Mously C; Moldofsky H. (1996). Periodic K-alpha sleep EEG activity and periodic limb movements during sleep: Comparisons of clinical features and sleep parameters. *Sleep* 19(3):200-204.

Mahowald MW; Mahowald ML; Bundlie SR; Ytterberg SR. (1989). Sleep fragmentation in rheumatoid arthritis. *Arthritis and Rheumatism* 32:974-983.

Moldofsky H. (1989). Sleep and fibrositis syndrome. *Rheumatic Disease Clinics of North America* 15:91-103.

Moldofsky H; Scarisbrick P. (1976). Induction of neurasthenic musculoeskeletal pain syndrome by selective sleep stage deprivation. *Psychosomatic Medicine* 38:35-44.

Moldofsky H; Scarisbrick P; England R; Smythe H. (1975). Musculoskeletal symptoms and non-REM sleep disturbance in patients with "fibrositis syndrome" and healthy subjects. *Psychosomatic Medicine* 37:341-351.

Molony RR; MacPeek DM; Schiffman PL; Frank M; Neubauer JA; Schwartzberg M; Seibold JR. (1986). Sleep, sleep apnea, and fibromyalgia syndrome. *Journal of Rheumatology* 13:797-800.

Older SA; Battafarano DF; Danning CL; Ward JA; Grady EP; Derman S; Russell IJ. (1998). The effects of delta wave sleep interruption on pain thresholds and fibromyalgia-like symptoms in healthy subjects: Correlations with insulin-like growth factor I. *Journal of Rheumatology* 25(6):1180-1186.

Paiva T; Batista A; Martins P; Martins A. (1995). The relationship between headaches and sleep disturbances. *Headache* 35(10):590-596.

Perlis ML; Giles DE; Bootzin RR; Dikman ZV; Fleming GM; Drummond SP; Rose MW. (1997). Alpha sleep and information processing, perception of sleep, pain, and arousability in fibromyalgia. *International Journal of Neurosciences* 89 (3-4):265-280.

Phillips GD; Cousins MJ. (1986). Neurological mechanisms of pain and the relationship of pain, anxiety, and sleep. In Cousins MJ; Phillips GD, eds. *Acute pain management*. New York: Churchill Livingstone; pp. 21-48.

Pilowski I; Crettenden I; Townly M. (1985). Sleep disturbance in pain clinic patients. *Pain* 23:27-33.

Reilly PA; Littlejohn GO. (1993). Diurnal variation in symptoms and signs of the fibromyalgia syndrome (FS). *Journal of Musculoskeletal Pain* 1:237-243.

Roizenblatt S; Moldofsky H; Benedito-Silva AA; Tufik S. (2001). Alpha sleep characteristics in fibromyalgia. *Arthritis and Rheumatism* 44(1):222-230.

Roizenblatt S; Tufik S; Goldenberg J; Pinto LR; Feldman DP. (1997). Juvenile fibromyalgia: clinical and polysomnographic aspects. *Journal of Rheumatology* 24:579-585.

Schaefer KM. (1995). Sleep disturbance and fatigue in women with fibromyalgia and chronic fatigue syndrome. *Journal of Obstetrics, Gynecology and Neonatal Nursing* 24:229-233.

Scharf MB; Hauck M; Stover R; McDannold M; Berkowitz D. (1998). Effect of gamma-hydroxybutyrate on pain, fatigue, and the alpha sleep anomaly in patients with fibromyalgia. Preliminary report. *Journal of Rheumatology* 25(10): 1986-1990.

Sergi M; Rizzi M; Braghiroli A; Puttini PS; Greco M; Cazzola M; Andreoli A. (1999). Periodic breathing during sleep in patients affected by fibromyalgia syndrome. *European Respiration Journal* 14(1):203-208.

Shaver JL; Lentz M; Landis CA; Heitkemper MM; Buchwald DS; Woods NF. (1997). Sleep, psychological distress, and stress arousal in women with fibromyalgia. *Research in Nursing and Health* 20(3):247-257.

Smythe HA. (1995). Studies of sleep in fibromyalgia: Techniques, clinical significance, and future directions. *British Journal of Rheumatology* 34(10):897-899.

Smythe HA; Moldofsky H. (1977). Two contributions to understanding "fibrositis" syndrome. *Bulletin of Rheumatic Diseases* 28:928-931.

Staedt J; Windt H; Hajaki G; Stoppe G; Rudolph G; Ensink FBM. (1993). Cluster arousal analysis in chronic pain-disturbed sleep. *Journal of Sleep Research* 2:134-137.

Tishler M; Barak Y; Paran D; Yaron M. (1997). Sleep disturbances, fibromyalgia and primary Sjogren's syndrome. *Clinical and Experimental Rheumatology* 15(1):71-74.

Touchon J. (1995). [Use of antidepressants in sleep disorders: Practical considerations] Utilisation des antidepresseurs dans les troubles du sommeil: Considerations pratiques. *Encephale* 21 Spec. No. 7:41-747.

Touchon J; Besset A; Billiard M; Simon L; Herrison C; Cadihac J. (1988). Fibrositis syndrome: Polysomnographic and psychological aspects. In Koella WP; Obai F; Schulz H; Visser P, eds. *Sleep '86.* New York: Gustav Fischer Verlag: pp. 445-447.

Walsh JK; Hartman PG; Schweitzer PK. (1994). Slow wave sleep deprivation and waking function. *Journal of Sleep Research* 3:16-25.

Ware JC; Russell IJ; Campos E. (1986). Alpha intrusions into the sleep of depression and fibromyalgia syndrome (fibrositis) patients. *Sleep Research* 15:210.

Wittig RM; Zorick FJ; Blumer D; Heilbronn M; Roth T. (1982). Disturbed sleep in patients complaning of chronic pain. *Journal of Nerve and Mental Diseases* 170:429-431.

Wolfe F; Cathey MA. (1983). Prevalence of primary and secondary fibrositis. *Journal of Rheumatology* 10:965-968.

Wolfe F; Smythe HA; Yunus MB; Bennett RM; Bombardier C; Goldenberg DL; Tugwell P; Campbell SM; Abeles M; Clark P. (1990). The American College of Rheumatology 1990 criteria for the classification of fibromyalgia: Report of the multicenter criteria committee. *Arthritis and Rheumatism* 33:160-172.

Yunus MB; Aldag JC. (1996). Restless legs syndrome and leg cramps in fibromyalgia syndrome: A controlled study. *British Medical Journal* 312(7042):1339.

Yunus MB; Masi AT; Calabro JJ; Miller KA; Feigenbaum SI. (1981). Primary fibromyalgia (fibrositis): Clinical study of 50 patients with matched controls. *Seminars in Arthritis and Rheumatism* 11:151-172.

*Smoking*

Aaron LA; Buchwald D. (2000). Tobacco use and chronic fatigue syndrome, fibromyalgia, and temporomandibular disorder. *Archives of Internal Medicine* 160(15):2398-2401.

Jay SJ. (2000). Tobacco use and chronic fatigue syndrome, fibromyalgia, and temporomandibular disorder. *Archives of Internal Medicine* 160(15):2398-2401.

Kurtze N; Gundersen KT; Svebak S. (1998). The role of anxiety and depression in fatigue and patterns of pain among subgroups of fibromyalgia patients. *British Journal of Medical Psychology* 71 (Pt. 2):185-194.

Kurtze N; Gundersen KT; Svebak S. (1999). Quality of life, functional disability and lifestyle among subgroups of fibromyalgia patients: The significance of anxiety and depression. *British Journal of Medical Psychology* 72(Pt. 4):471-484.
Ostensen M; Schei B. (1997). Sociodemographic characteristics and gynecological disease in 40-42 year old women reporting musculoskeletal disease. *Scandinavian Journal of Rheumatology* 26(6):426-434.

## Social Networks

Bolwijn PH; van Santen-Hoeufft MH; Baars HM; Kaplan CD; van der Linden S. (1996). The social network characteristics of fibromyalgia patients compared with healthy controls. *Arthritis Care Research* 9(1):18-26.

## Sphenopalatine Blocks

Janzen VD; Scudds R. (1997). Sphenopalatine blocks in the treatment of pain in fibromyalgia and myofascial pain syndrome. *Laryngoscope* 107(10):1420-1422.

## Spinal Tracts

Mense S. (1998). Descending antinociception and fibromyalgia. *Zeitschrift Rheumatologie* 57 (Suppl. 2):23-26.
Mense S. (2000). Neurobiological concepts of fibromyalgia—the possible role of descending spinal tracts. *Scandinavian Journal of Rheumatology* (Suppl. 113): 24-29.

## Staphylococcus *Toxoid Vaccine*

Andersson M; Bagby JR; Dyrehag L; Gottfries C. (1998). Effects of staphylococcus toxoid vaccine on pain and fatigue in patients with fibromyalgia/chronic fatigue syndrome. *European Journal of Pain* 2(2):133-142.

## Substance P

Evengard B; Nilsson CG; Lindh G; Lindquist L; Eneroth P; Fredrikson S; Terenius L; Henriksson KG. (1998). Chronic fatigue syndrome differs from fibromyalgia. No evidence for elevated substance P levels in cerebrospinal fluid of patients with chronic fatigue syndrome. *Pain* 78(2):153-155.
Larson AA; Giovengo SL; Russell IJ; Michalek JE. (2000). Changes in the concentrations of amino acids in the cerebrospinal fluid that correlate with pain in patients with fibromyalgia: Implications for nitric oxide pathways. *Pain* 87(2): 201-211.

Liu Z; Welin M; Bragee B; Nyberg F. (2000). A high-recovery extraction procedure for quantitative analysis of substance P and opioid peptides in human cerebrospinal fluid. *Peptides* 21(6):853-860.

Pongratz DE; Sievers M. (2000). Fibromyalgia-symptom or diagnosis: A definition of the position. *Scandinavian Journal of Rheumatology* (Suppl. 113):3-7.

Schwarz MJ; Spath M; Muller-Bardorff H; Pongratz DE; Bondy B; Ackenheil M. (1999). Relationship of substance P, 5-hydroxyindole acetic acid and tryptophan in serum of fibromyalgia patients. *Neurosciences Letters* 259(3):196-198.

Sprott H; Bradley LA; Oh SJ; Wintersberger W; Alarcon GS; Mussell HG; Tseng A; Gay RE; Gay S. (1998). Immunohistochemical and molecular studies of serotonin, substance P, galanin, pituitary adenylyl cyclase-activating polypeptide, and secretoneurin in fibromyalgic muscle tissue. *Arthritis and Rheumatism* 41(9):1689-1694.

## Super Malic

Russell IJ; Michalek JE; Flechas JD; Abraham GE. (1995). Treatment of fibromyalgia syndrome with Super Malic: A randomized, double blind, placebo controlled, crossover pilot study. *Journal of Rheumatology* 22(5):953-958.

## Surgeries

ter Borg EJ; Gerards-Rociu E; Haanen HC; Westers P. (1999). High frequency of hysterectomies and appendectomies in fibromyalgia compared with rheumatoid arthritis: A pilot study. *Clinical Rheumatology* 18(1):1-3.

Wagener P; Hein R; Felstehausen KH. (1997). [Gynecologic operations in fibromyalgia syndrome. A retrospective analysis of 890 patients of a rheumatologic and general practice] Gynakologische operationen beim fibromyalgiesyndrom. Eine retrospektive analyse an 890 patientinnen einer rheumatologischen und einer allgemeinpraxis. *Fortschrift Medizin* 115(24):39-40.

## Systemic Lupus Erythematosus

Abu-Shakra M; Mader R; Langevitz P; Friger M; Codish S; Neumann L; Buskila D. (1999). Quality of life in systemic lupus erythematosus: A controlled study. *Journal of Rheumatology* 26(2):306-309.

Akkasilpa S; Minor M; Goldman D; Magder LS; Petri M. (2000). Association of coping responses with fibromyalgia tender points in patients with systemic lupus erythematosus. *Journal of Rheumatology* 27(3):671-674.

Bennett R. (1997). The concurrence of lupus and fibromyalgia: Implications for diagnosis and management. *Lupus* 6(6):494-499.

Bruce IN; Mak VC; Hallett DC; Gladman DD; Urowitz MB. (1999). Factors associated with fatigue in patients with systemic lupus erythematosus. *Annals of Rheumatic Diseases* 58(6):379-381.

Calvo-Alen J; Bastian HM; Straaton KV; Burgard SL; Mikhail IS; Alarcon GS. (1995). Identification of patient subsets among those presumptively diagnosed with, referred, and/or followed up for systemic lupus erythematosus at a large tertiary care center. *Arthritis and Rheumatism* 38(10):1475-1484.

Da Costa D; Dobkin PL; Fitzcharles MA; Fortin PR; Beaulieu A; Zummer M; Senecal JL; Goulet JR; Rich E; Choquette D; Clarke AE. (2000). Determinants of health status in fibromyalgia: A comparative study with systemic lupus erythematosus. *Journal of Rheumatology* 27(2):365-372.

Gladman DD; Urowitz MB; Gough J; MacKinnon A. (1997). Fibromyalgia is a major contributor to quality of life in lupus. *Journal of Rheumatology* 24(11):2145-2148.

Gladman DD; Urowitz MB; Slonim D; Glanz B; Carlen P; Noldy N; Gough J; Pauzner R; Heslegrave R; Darby P; MacKinnon A. (2000). Evaluation of predictive factors for neurocognitive dysfunction in patients with inactive systemic lupus erythematosus. *Journal of Rheumatology* 27(10):2367-2371.

Godfrey T; Khamashta MA; Hughes GR. (1998). Therapeutic advances in systemic lupus erythematosus. *Current Opinions in Rheumatology* 10(5):435-441.

Grafe A; Wollina U; Tebbe B; Sprott H; Uhlemann C; Hein G. (1999). Fibromyalgia in lupus erythematosus. *Acta Dermatologica Venereologica* 79(1):62-64.

Handa R; Aggarwal P; Wali JP; Wig N; Dwivedi SN. (1998). Fibromyalgia in Indian patients with SLE. *Lupus* 7(7):475-478.

Lopez-Osa A; Jimenez-Alonso J; Garcia-Sanchez A; Sanchez-Tapia C; Perez M; Peralta MI; Gutierrez-Cabello F; Morente G. (1999). Fibromyalgia in Spanish patients with systemic lupus erythematosus. *Lupus* 8(4):332-333.

Petri M. (1995). Clinical features of systemic lupus erythematosus. *Current Opinions in Rheumatology* 7(5):395-401.

Romano TJ. (1995). Fibromyalgia prevalence in patients with systemic lupus erythematosus: Comment on the article by Middleton et al. *Arthritis and Rheumatism* 38(6):872.

Romano TJ. (1997). Possible concomitant fibromyalgia in systemic lupus erythematosus patients with overt central nervous system disease but with cognitive deficits: Comment on the article by Kozora et al. *Arthritis and Rheumatism* 40(8):1544-1545.

Taylor J; Skan J; Erb N; Carruthers D; Bowman S; Gordon C; Isenberg D. (2000). Lupus patients with fatigue—is there a link with fibromyalgia syndrome? *Rheumatology* (Oxford) 39(6):620-623.

Wallace DJ. (1995). Prevalence of fibromyalgia in systemic lupus erythematosus patients: Comment on the article by Middleton et al. *Arthritis and Rheumatism* 38(6):872.

Wang B; Gladman DD; Urowitz MB. (1998). Fatigue in lupus is not correlated with disease activity. *Journal of Rheumatology* 25(5):892-895.

### *Temporomandibular Disorder*

Aaron LA; Burke MM; Buchwald D. (2000). Overlapping conditions among patients with chronic fatigue syndrome, fibromyalgia, and temporomandibular disorder. *Archives of Internal Medicine* 160(2):221-227.

Auvenshine RC. (1997). Psychoneuroimmunology and its relationship to the differential diagnosis of temporomandibular disorders. *Dentistry Clinics of North America* 41(2):279-296.

De Laat A. (1997). [Etiologic factors in temporomandibular joint disorders and pain] Facteurs etiologiques dans les troubles et l'algie temporo-mandibulaires. *Revue Belge de Medicine Dentale* 52(4):115-123.

Hedenberg-Magnusson B; Ernberg M; Kopp S. (1997). Symptoms and signs of temporomandibular disorders in patients with fibromyalgia and local myalgia of the temporomandibular system. A comparative study. *Acta Odontologica Scandinavica* 55(6):344-349.

Hedenberg-Magnusson B; Ernberg M; Kopp S. (1999). Presence of orofacial pain and temporomandibular disorder in fibromyalgia. A study by questionnaire. *Swedish Dentistry Journal* 23(5-6):185-192.

Kashima K; Rahman OI; Sakoda S; Shiba R. (1999). Increased pain sensitivity of the upper extremities of TMD patients with myalgia to experimentally-evoked noxious stimulation: Possibility of worsened endogenous opioid systems. *Cranio* 17(4):241-246.

Korszun A; Papadopoulos E; Demitrack M; Engleberg C; Crofford L. (1998). The relationship between temporomandibular disorders and stress-associated syndromes. *Oral Surgery, Oral Medicine, Oral Pathology, Oral Radiology and Endodontics* 86(4):416-420.

Miller VJ; Zeltser R; Yoeli Z; Bodner L. (1997). Ehlers-Danlos syndrome, fibromyalgia and temporomandibular disorder: Report of an unusual combination. *Cranio* 15(3):267-269.

Pennacchio EA; Borg-Stein J; Keith DA. (1998). The incidence of pain in the muscles of mastication in patients with fibromyalgia. *Journal of the Massachusetts Dental Society* 47(3):8-12.

Plesh O; Wolfe F; Lane N. (1996). The relationship between fibromyalgia and temporomandibular disorders: Prevalence and symptom severity. *Journal of Rheumatology* 23(11):1948-1952.

Stohler CS. (1999). Muscle-related temporomandibular disorders. *Journal of Orofacial Pain* 13(4):273-284.

Wright EF; Des Rosier KF; Clark MK; Bifano SL. (1997). Identifying undiagnosed rheumatic disorders among patients with TMD. *Journal of the American Dental Association* 128(6):738-744.

**Tender Point Pathophysiology**

Croft P; Burt J; Schollum J; Thomas E; Macfarlane G; Silman A. (1996). More pain, more tender points: Is fibromyalgia just one end of a continuous spectrum? *Annals of Rheumatic Diseases* 55(7):482-485.

Fassbender K; Samborsky W; Kellner M; Muller W; Lautenbacher S. (1997). Tender points, depressive and functional symptoms: Comparison between fibromyalgia and major depression. *Clinical Rheumatology* 16(1):76-79.

Hapidou EG; Rollman GB. (1998). Menstrual cycle modulation of tender points. *Pain* 77(2):151-161.

Jacobs JW; Rasker JJ; van der Heide A; Boersma JW; de Blecourt AC; Griep EN; van Rijswijk MH; Bijlsma JW. (1996). Lack of correlation between the mean tender point score and self-reported pain in fibromyalgia. *Arthritis Care Research* 9(2):105-111.

Jeschonneck M; Grohmann G; Hein G; Sprott H. (2000). Abnormal microcirculation and temperature in skin above tender points in patients with fibromyalgia. *Rheumatology* (Oxford) 39(8):917-921.

Kosek E; Ekholm J; Hansson P. (1995). Increased pressure pain sensibility in fibromyalgia patients is located deep to the skin but not restricted to muscle tissue. *Pain* 63(3):335-339.

McBeth J; Macfarlane GJ; Benjamin S; Morris S; Silman AJ. (1999). The association between tender points, psychological distress, and adverse childhood experiences: a community-based study. *Arthritis and Rheumatism* 42(7):1397-1404.

McIntosh MJ; Hewett JE; Buckelew SP; Conway RR; Rossy LA. (1998). Protocol for verifying expertise in locating fibromyalgia tender points. *Arthritis Care Research* 11(3):210-216.

Nicassio PM; Weisman MH; Schuman C; Young CW. (2000). The role of generalized pain and pain behavior in tender point scores in fibromyalgia. *Journal of Rheumatology* 27(4):1056-1062.

Okifuji A; Turk DC; Sinclair JD; Starz TW; Marcus DA. (1997). A standardized manual tender point survey. I. Development and determination of a threshold point for the identification of positive tender points in fibromyalgia syndrome. *Journal of Rheumatology* 24(2):377-383.

Quimby LG; Block SR; Gratwick GM. (1998). What use are fibromyalgia control points? *Journal of Rheumatology* 25(12):2476.

Rea T; Russo J; Katon W; Ashley RL; Buchwald D. (1999). A prospective study of tender points and fibromyalgia during and after an acute viral infection. *Archives of Internal Medicine* 159(8):865-870.

Sigal LH; Chang DJ; Sloan V. (1998). 18 tender points and the "18-wheeler" sign: Clues to the diagnosis of fibromyalgia. *Journal of the American Medical Association* 279(6):434.

Smythe H. (1998). Examination for tenderness: Learning to use 4 kg force. *Journal of Rheumatology* 25(1):149-151.

Sprott H; Jeschonneck M; Grohmann G; Hein G. (2000). [Microcirculatory changes over the tender points in fibromyalgia patients after acupuncture therapy (measured with laser-Doppler flowmetry)] Anderung der durchblutung uber den tender points bei fibromyalgie-patienten nach einer akupunkturtherapie (gemessen mit der laser-doppler-flowmetrie). *Wien Klinische Wochenschrift* 112(13):580-586.

Tunks E; McCain GA; Hart LE; Teasell RW; Goldsmith CH; Rollman GB; McDermid AJ; DeShane PJ. (1995). The reliability of examination for tenderness in patients with myofascial pain, chronic fibromyalgia and controls. *Journal of Rheumatology* 22(5):944-952.

Wolfe F. (1997). The relation between tender points and fibromyalgia symptom variables: Evidence that fibromyalgia is not a discrete disorder in the clinic. *Annals of Rheumatic Diseases* 56(4):268-271.

Wolfe F. (1998). What use are fibromyalgia control points? *Journal of Rheumatology* 25(3):546-550.

### *Thyroid Microsomal Antibodies*

Aarflot T; Bruusgaard D. (1996). Association between chronic widespread musculoskeletal complaints and thyroid autoimmunity. Results from a community survey. *Scandinavian Journal of Primary Health Care* 14(2):111-115.

### *Tramadol*

Biasi G; Manca S; Manganelli S; Marcolongo R. (1998). Tramadol in the fibromyalgia syndrome: A controlled clinical trial versus placebo. *International Journal of Clinical Pharmacology Research* 18(1):13-19.

Freye E; Levy J. (2000). Acute abstinence syndrome following abrupt cessation of long-term use of tramadol (Ultram(R)): A case study. *European Journal of Pain* 4(3):307-311.

### *Trauma*

Aaron LA; Bradley LA; Alarcon GS; Triana-Alexander M; Alexander RW; Martin MY; Alberts KR. (1997). Perceived physical and emotional trauma as precipitating events in fibromyalgia. Associations with health care seeking and disability status but not pain severity. *Arthritis and Rheumatism* 40(3):453-460.

Bohr T. (1995). A long-term follow-up on "post-traumatic fibromyalgia" patients. *American Journal of Physical Medicine and Rehabilitation* 74(6):476-477.

Buskila D; Neumann L; Vaisberg G; Alkalay D; Wolfe F. (1997). Increased rates of fibromyalgia following cervical spine injury. A controlled study of 161 cases of traumatic injury. *Arthritis and Rheumatism* 40(3):446-452.

Cohen ML; Quintner JL. (1998). Altered nociception, but not fibromyalgia, after cervical spine injury: Comment on the article by Buskila et al. *Arthritis and Rheumatism* 41(1):183-184.

Ferrari R; Kwan O. (1999). Fibromyalgia and physical and emotional trauma: How are they related? *Arthritis and Rheumatism* 42(4):828-830.

Ferrari R; Russell AS. (1998). Neck injury and chronic pain syndromes: Comment on the article by Buskila et al. *Arthritis and Rheumatism* 41(4):758-789.

Fishbain DA; Rosomoff HL. (1998). Posttraumatic fibromyalgia at pain facilities versus rheumatologists' offices: A commentary. *American Journal of Physical and Medical Rehabilitation* 77(6):562.

Gardner GC. (2000). Fibromyalgia following trauma: Psychology or biology? *Current Reviews on Pain* 4(4):295-300.

Gordon DA. (1997). The rheumatologist and chronic whiplash syndrome. *Journal of Rheumatology* 24(4):617-618.

Jenzer G. (1995). [Clinical aspects and neurologic expert assessment in sequelae of whiplash injury to the cervical spine] Klinische aspekte und neurologische begutachtung beim zustand nach beschleunigungsmechanismus an der halswirbelsaule. *Nervenarzt* 66(10):730-735.

Link R; Balint G; Pavlik G; Otto J; Krause W. (1996). [Topical treatment of soft tissue rheumatism and athletic injuries. Effectiveness and tolerance of a new ketoprofen gel] Topische behandlung von weichteilrheumatismus und sportverletzungen. wirksamkeit und vertraglichkeit eines neuen ketoprofengels. *Fortschrift Medizin* 114(25):311-314.

Nonarticular rheumatism, sports-related injuries, and related conditions. (1997). *Current Opinions in Rheumatology* 9(2):B42-B65.

Pinals RS. (1997). Nonarticular rheumatism, sports-related injuries, and related conditions. *Current Opinions in Rheumatology* 9(2):133-134.

Smith MD. (1998). Relationship of fibromyalgia to site and type of trauma: Comment on the articles by Buskila et al. and Aaron et al. *Arthritis and Rheumatism* 41(2):378-379.

White KP; Carette S; Harth M; Teasell RW. (2000). Trauma and fibromyalgia: Is there an association and what does it mean? *Seminars in Arthritis and Rheumatism* 29(4):200-216.

White KP; Ostbye T; Harth M; Nielson W; Speechley M; Teasell R; Bourne R. (2000). Perspectives on posttraumatic fibromyalgia: a random survey of Canadian general practitioners, orthopedists, physiatrists, and rheumatologists. *Journal of Rheumatology* 27(3):790-796.

Wigley RD. (1998). Can accident or occupation cause fibromyalgia? *New Zealand Medical Journal* 27;111(1060):60.

*Treatment*

Akama H. (2000). Management of fibromyalgia. *Annals of Internal Medicine* 132(12):1005.

Alarcon GS; Bradley LA. (1998). Advances in the treatment of fibromyalgia: Current status and future directions. *American Journal of Medical Sciences* 315(6): 397-404.

Bakker C; Rutten M; van Santen-Hoeufft M; Bolwijn P; van Doorslaer E; Bennett K; van der Linden S. (1995). Patient utilities in fibromyalgia and the association with other outcome measures. *Journal of Rheumatology* 22(8):1536-1543.

Bennett RM. (1995). Fibromyalgia: The commonest cause of widespread pain. *Comprehensive Therapy* 21(6):269-75.

Bennett RM. (1996). Multidisciplinary group programs to treat fibromyalgia patients. *Rheumatic Diseases Clinics of North America* 22(2):351-367.

Bennett RM; Burckhardt CS; Clark SR; O'Reilly CA; Wiens AN; Campbell SM. (1996). Group treatment of fibromyalgia: A 6 month outpatient program. *Journal of Rheumatology* 23(3):521-528.

Burckhardt CS; Jones KD; Clark SR. (1998). Soft tissue problems associated with rheumatic disease. *Lippincotts Primary Care Practice* 2(1):20-29; quiz 30-31.

Buskila D. (1999). Drug therapy. *Baillieres Best Practice Research in Clinical Rheumatology* 13(3):479-485.

Clauw DJ. (2000). Treating fibromyalgia: Science vs. art. *American Family Physician* 62(7):1492, 1494.

Cohn LJ. (2000). Management of fibromyalgia. *Annals of Internal Medicine* 132(12):1005.

Eisinger J; Dupond JL. (1996). [Should patients with fibromyalgia be doped?] Faut-il doper les fibromyalgiques? *Revue Medicine Interne* 17(12):977-978.

Finckh A; Morabia A; Deluze C; Vischer T. (1998). Validation of questionnaire-based response criteria of treatment efficacy in the fibromyalgia syndrome. *Arthritis Care Research* 11(2):116-123.

Hewett JE; Buckelew SP; Johnson JC; Shaw SE; Huyser B; Fu YZ. (1995). Selection of measures suitable for evaluating change in fibromyalgia clinical trials. *Journal of Rheumatology* 22(12):2307-2312.

Huppert A. (2000). Management of fibromyalgia. *Annals of Internal Medicine* 132(12):1004; discussion 1005.

Keel P. (1999). Pain management strategies and team approach. *Baillieres Best Practice Research in Clinical Rheumatology* 13(3):493-506.

Keel PJ; Bodoky C; Gerhard U; Muller W. (1998). Comparison of integrated group therapy and group relaxation training for fibromyalgia. *Clinical Journal of Pain* 14(3):232-238.

Lamberg L. (1999). Patients in pain need round-the-clock care. *Journal of the American Medical Association* 281(8):689-690.

Langer HE. (1995). [Patient education—A contribution to improvement of long-term management of patients with rheumatism] Patientenschulung—Ein beitrag zur verbesserung der langzeitbetreuung von rheumapatienten. *Zeitschrift Rheumatologie* 54(4):207-212.

Leventhal LJ. (1999). Management of fibromyalgia. *Annals of Internal Medicine* 131(11):850-858.

Littlejohn G. (1995). The fibromyalgia syndrome. Outcome is good with minimal intervention. *British Medical Journal* 310(6991):1406.

Lloyd R. (2000). How should we manage fibromyalgia? *Annals of Rheumatic Diseases* 59(6):490.

Louis R; Repellin F; Louis C. (1998). [Surgery for lumbago and fibromyalgia] Chirurgie des lombalgies et fibromyalgie. *Acta Orthopedica Belgica* 64 (Suppl. 2):53-56.

Mason LW; Goolkasian P; McCain GA. (1998). Evaluation of multimodal treatment program for fibromyalgia. *Journal of Behavioral Medicine* 21(2):163-178.

McCain GA. (1996). A cost-effective approach to the diagnosis and treatment of fibromyalgia. *Rheumatic Diseases Clinics of North America* 22(2):323-349.

Millea PJ; Holloway RL. (2000). Treating fibromyalgia. *American Family Physician* 62(7):1575-1582, 1587.

Muilenburg N. (2000). Management of fibromyalgia. *Annals of Internal Medicine* 132(12):1004-1005; discussion 1005.

Muller W; Pongratz D; Barlin E; Eich W; Farber L; Haus U; Lautenschlager J; Mense S; Neeck G; Offenbacher M; Spath M; Stratz T; Tolk J; Welzel D; Wiech K; Wohlgemuth M. (2000). The challenge of fibromyalgia: New approaches. *Scandinavian Journal of Rheumatology* (Suppl. 113):86.

Parziale JR. (1999). The clinical management of fibromyalgia. *Medical Health of Rhode Island* 82(9):325-328.

Reilly PA. (1999). How should we manage fibromyalgia? *Annals of Rheumatic Diseases* 58(6):325-326.

Richards S; Cleare A. (2000). Treating fibromyalgia. *Rheumatology* (Oxford) 39(4): 343-346.

Rossy LA; Buckelew SP; Dorr N; Hagglund KJ; Thayer JF; McIntosh MJ; Hewett JE; Johnson JC. (1999). A meta-analysis of fibromyalgia treatment interventions. *Annals of Behavioral Medicine* 21(2):180-191.

Russell IJ. (1996). Fibromyalgia syndrome: Approaches to management. *Bulletin of Rheumatic Diseases* 45(3):1-4.

Rutten-van Molken MP; Bakker CH; van Doorslaer EK; van der Linden S. (1995). Methodological issues of patient utility measurement. Experience from two clinical trials. *Medical Care* 33(9):922-937.

Sandstrom MJ; Keefe FJ. (1998). Self-management of fibromyalgia: The role of formal coping skills training and physical exercise training programs. *Arthritis Care Research* 11(6):432-447.

Schachna L; Littlejohn G. (1999). Primary care and specialist management options. *Baillieres Best Practice Research in Clinical Rheumatology* 13(3):469-477.

Sim J; Adams N. (1999). Physical and other non-pharmacological interventions for fibromyalgia. *Baillieres Best Practice Research in Clinical Rheumatology* 13(3):507-523.

Strobel ES; Wild J; Muller W. (1998). [Interdisciplinary group therapy for fibromyalgia] Interdisziplinare gruppentherapie fur die fibromyalgie. *Zeitschrift Rheumatologie* 57(2):89-94.

Tanum L; Malt UF. (1995). Sodium lactate infusion in fibromyalgia patients. *Biological Psychiatry* 38(8):559-561.

Thomas E; Ginies P; Blotman F. (1999). Fibromyalgia as a national issue: The French example. *Baillieres Best Practice Research in Clinical Rheumatology* 13(3):525-529.

Turk DC; Okifuji A; Sinclair JD; Starz TW. (1998). Interdisciplinary treatment for fibromyalgia syndrome: Clinical and statistical significance. *Arthritis Care Research* 11(3):186-195.

White KP; Harth M. (1996). An analytical review of 24 controlled clinical trials for fibromyalgia syndrome (FMS). *Pain* 64(2):211-219.

Wolfe F. (1995). The epidemiology of drug treatment failure in rheumatoid arthritis. *Baillieres Clinical Rheumatology* 9(4):619-632.

Wolfe F. (2000). Management of fibromyalgia. *Annals of Internal Medicine* 132(12):1004; discussion 1005.

Zborovskii AB; Babaeva AR. (1996). [New trends in the study of the primary fibromyalgic syndrome] Novye napravleniia v izuchenii sindroma pervichnoi fibromialgii. *Vestn Ross Akad Med Nauk* (11):52-56.

Zucker DR; Schmid CH; McIntosh MW; D'Agostino RB; Selker HP; Lau J. (1997). Combining single patient (N-of-1) trials to estimate population treatment effects and to evaluate individual patient responses to treatment. *Journal of Clinical Epidemiology* 50(4):401-410.

*Trigger Points*

Borg-Stein J; Stein J. (1996). Trigger points and tender points: One and the same? Does injection treatment help? *Rheumatic Diseases Clinics of North America* 22(2):305-322.

Hong CZ; Hsueh TC. (1996). Difference in pain relief after trigger point injections in myofascial pain patients with and without fibromyalgia. *Archives of Physical and Medical Rehabilitation* 77(11):1161-1166.

Jayson MI. (1996). Fibromyalgia and trigger point injections. *Bulletin of Hospital Joint Disease* 55(4):176-177.

Potter PJ. (1997). Trigger point injections. *Archives of Physical and Medical Rehabilitation* 78(6):676.

Schneider MJ. (1995). Tender points/fibromyalgia vs. trigger points/myofascial pain syndrome: A need for clarity in terminology and differential diagnosis. *Journal of Manipulative Physiology Therapy* 18(6):398-406.

## Tryptophan

Birdsall TC. (1998). 5-Hydroxytryptophan: A clinically-effective serotonin precursor. *Alternative Medicine Reviews* 3(4):271-280.

Schwarz MJ; Spath M; Muller-Bardorff H; Pongratz DE; Bondy B; Ackenheil M. (1999). Relationship of substance P, 5-hydroxyindole acetic acid and tryptophan in serum of fibromyalgia patients. *Neurosciences Letters* 259(3):196-198.

## Urine

Xie X; Yang Q; Zhang J; Tan Y; Li X; Liu Y. (1998). [Relation between fibromyalgia and bacterial urine]. *Hunan I Ko Ta Hsueh Hsueh Pao* 23(2):217.

## Venlafaxine

Dryson E. (2000). Venlafaxine and fibromyalgia. *New Zealand Medical Journal* 113(1105):87.

Dwight MM; Arnold LM; O'Brien H; Metzger R; Morris-Park E; Keck PE Jr. (1998). An open clinical trial of venlafaxine treatment of fibromyalgia. *Psychosomatics* 39(1):14-17.

## Virology

Buchwald D; Ashley RL; Pearlman T; Kith P; Komaroff AL. (1996). Viral serologies in patients with chronic fatigue and chronic fatigue syndrome. *Journal of Medical Virology* 50(1):25-30.

## Weather

Quick DC. (1997). Joint pain and weather. A critical review of the literature. *Minnesota Medicine* 80(3):25-29.

## Zolpidem

Moldofsky H; Lue FA; Mously C; Roth-Schechter B; Reynolds WJ. (1996). The effect of zolpidem in patients with fibromyalgia: A dose ranging, double blind, placebo controlled, modified crossover study. *Journal of Rheumatology* 23(3):529-533.

Rothschild BM. (1997). Zolpidem efficacy in fibromyalgia. *Journal of Rheumatology* 24(5):1012-1013.

# Index

5-HT3-receptor, 84-85
5-hydroxyindolacetic acid (5-HIAA), 89-90
5-hydroxytrytophan (5-HTP), 96
IGF-1, 39, 43, 50-51
P450IID6 oxidative enzyme, 26
T102 allele, 85

Aarflot, T., 93
Aaron, L.A., 79, 94
Abuse, 1
Acasuso-Diaz, M., 53
Acetaminophen, 69
Acupuncture, 2-3, 5
Acute fatigue, 36
Acute pain, 71
Adenosine 3'5'-phosphate phosphodiesterase, cyclic, 33
Adenovirus, 97
Adler, G.K., 66
Adrenal androgens, hyposecretion of, 26
Adrenocorticotropic hormone (ACTH), 59, 65
Adult growth hormone deficiency, 50
Aerobic endurance, 35
Affective distress and anxiety, 3
Agargun, M.Y., 72
Agents, chemical intolerance, 17
Aging, 4
Akinetic syndrome, 59
Akkasilpa, S., 24, 91
Alcohol, 4
Alexander, R.W., 1
Allergy, 4, 49-50
Allodynia, 83
Aloe, 4-5
*Aloe vera* gel, 4-5
Alpha anomaly, 41, 87
Alpha-adrenergic dominance, 33

Alternative medicine, 5
Ambrogio, N., 64
American College of Rheumatology, criteria for fibromyalgia, 37, 38
  and acetaminophen use, 69
  and Behcet's syndrome, 12
  and disability, 30
  and epidemiology, 33
  and fatigue, 91
  and fibromyalgia diagnosis, 48, 53
  and hyperkalemic periodic paralysis, 48
  and joint hypermobility, 53
American Pain Society, 62
Amir, M., 77
Amitriptyline, 6, 83
Ammer, K., 58
Amyotrophic lateral sclerosis, 73
ANA-negative children, 11
ANA-positive children, 11
Anderberg, U.M., 1, 68
Ankylosing spondylitis, 25
Anthraquinones, 5
Antibodies, 6-10
Anti-B2GPI antibodies, 8
Anticardiolipin antibody, 6-7
Antidepressants, 7, 79, 88, 97
Antiganglioside antibodies, 9-10, 43
Antinuclear antibody (ANA), 8, 11, 49
Antiphospholipid antibodies, 8-9, 10, 43
Antipolymer antibodies, 9
Anti-Sa, 11
Antiserotonin antibodies, 9-10, 43
Anxiety, 3, 15, 42
Ardicoglu, O., 15
Arnold, L.M., 7
Arthralgias, absence of and EMS, 31
Arthritis, rheumatoid, 1, 9, 14, 25, 27
Arthritis Impact Measurement Scales, 28